HEALING YOGA

for people living with cancer

HEALING YOGA

for people living with cancer

LISA HOLTBY

photographs by debra ragatz-paduano

TAYLOR TRADE PUBLISHING

Lanham NewYork Dallas Boulder Toronto Oxford

Published by Taylor Trade Publishing
An imprint of The Rowman & Littlefield Publishing Group, Inc.
4501 Forbes Boulevard, Suite 200
Lanham, Maryland 20706

Distributed by National Book Network

Any user of this exercise program assumes the risk of injury from performing the exercises. To reduce risk of injury, consult your physician before beginning this exercise program. The instructions and advice presented are in no way intended as a substitute for medical counseling. The creators and publishers of this program disclaim any liabilities or loss in connection with the exercise and advice herein.

Library of Congress Cataloging-in-Publication Data

Holtby, Lisa.
  Healing yoga for people living with cancer / Lisa Holtby.—1st Taylor Trade Pub. ed.
    p. cm.
  Includes bibliographical references.
  ISBN 1-58979-105-3 (pbk. : alk. paper)
  1. Yoga—Therapeutic use. 2. Cancer—Palliative treatment. I. Title.
  RC271.Y63H65 2004
  613.7'047—dc22

                        2004005990

∞   The paper used in this publication meets the minimum requirements of American National Standard for Information Sciences—Permanence of Paper for Printed Library Materials, ANSI/NISO Z39.48–1992.
Manufactured in the United States of America.

CONTENTS

ACKNOWLEDGMENTS

I wish to honor my agent, Linda Konner, for her perseverance; the founder of Anusara Yoga, John Friend, for his genius; the founder of Seattle Yoga Arts, Denise Benitez, for her leadership; Cancer Lifeline's Executive Director, Barbara Frederick, for her vision; my Landmark Education instructors, for their coaching; our incomparable nanny, Shelly Fayette, for her *joie de vivre*; and especially my guys, David and Benjamin Hlavsa, for making my life so sweet.

So many people contributed to the process of developing this book. Many thanks to photographer Debra Paduano, stylist Michelle Marshall, my Cancer Lifeline and Seattle Yoga Arts students, to Kathie Deviny, Laura Eastman, Judy Ellis, Ellen Forney, David Latourell, Ann Pelo, Robin Rivers, and Julie Walwick.

I especially appreciate the expertise of the physicians and yoga teachers who reviewed sections of this manuscript for accuracy:

Anthony Back, M.D., University of Washington, Cancer Lifeline Medical Advisory Group

Claire Barnett, M.D.

Denise Benitez, Certified Anusara Yoga Instructor

Raleigh A. Bowden, M.D.

Denise Carrico, Certified Integral Yoga teacher, Cancer Lifeline

Barbara Frederick, Executive Director, Cancer Lifeline

Betsy Gilbert, Assistant Training Coordinator, National Cancer Institute's Cancer Information Service

Sarahjoy Marsh, Certified Anusara Yoga Instructor

Stephen Smith, M.D., Group Health Cooperative

Lisa Talbott, M.P.H., Health Promotion Program Manager, Cancer Lifeline

FOREWORD

by Dr. Lee Hartwell, President and Director
and Dr. Alan Kristal, Division of Public Health Sciences

FRED HUTCHINSON CANCER RESEARCH CENTER
Seattle, Washington

Research over the past decade has brought enormous advances in our understanding of cancer. For example, we now know that cancer is the result of cells losing control of their own growth, and we know a great deal about genetic and behavioral factors that can increase or decrease cancer risk. There have also been significant changes in cancer treatment.

As a result of improved cancer screening techniques, such as mammography, we now diagnose cancer earlier, when it can be treated more effectively. And treatments themselves have changed: many are less invasive, have fewer side effects, and are more likely to lead to cure. More and more people are surviving cancer, and there is a new emphasis on helping those treated for cancer return to active, productive lives. Surgery, chemotherapy, or radiation treatments to treat cancer are difficult, but throughout and after treatment it is important to focus on increasing mobility, decreasing pain, and getting back to feeling good.

We are excited about the potential for yoga to help people with cancer. Practicing yoga can help restore range of motion, relieve tension, and bring a sense of calm and well-being into one's life. In addition, regular practice can help control the pain and discomfort that is often associated with cancer treatment. For people who were never physically active, yoga offers a new way to learn about and be comfortable in their bodies. For people who were active before their cancer treatment, yoga offers a return to physical activity that is intelligent, progressive, and respectful.

The author of this book, Lisa Holtby, has taught yoga since 1993 and spent two years teaching yoga to people recovering from cancer treatments. This book is based on her experience and insights into how yoga can assist cancer recovery. Lisa has also supported cancer research as the founder of Positive Yoga, an all-volunteer benefit for breast cancer research that she started in Seattle in 1997 that has since raised $230,000 and expanded to forty cities nationally.

As cancer researchers, our goal is to understand the basic biology of cancer, to create better treatments, and to develop public health programs that can prevent cancer from ever developing. We appreciate this book as a contribution to our shared goal, which is to decrease the human suffering caused by cancer.

welcome

Dear Reader:

Welcome! *Healing Yoga for People Living with Cancer* is based on my two years of teaching yoga classes for Cancer Lifeline* and is a compilation of my students' favorite sequences. I sincerely hope that the book is helpful to you in your journey. Even if you've never done yoga before, *Healing Yoga* is laid out so that you can easily follow along, just as if we were in class together. It is a way for you to actively participate in your own healing process. At any stage of living with cancer, practicing *Healing Yoga* will strengthen your own sense of well-being, comfort, and peace.

I know from personal experience how Healing Yoga helps during times of illness, grief, and fear. At the end of my second trimester of pregnancy, I was hospitalized for seven weeks due to life-threatening complications to my baby and me. I know what it is like to endure sickness and exhaustion for months on end, to be on heavy drugs, to feel like a pincushion from all the needle sticks of IVs, blood draws, and a PICC line, to depend completely on the competency of the medical staff taking care of me, to surrender my privacy, and to forgo my identity as a capable adult with a career and a home.

As a patient, paradoxically I was at my most vulnerable just when I needed to educate myself about my latest condition and advocate strongly for my son and myself. Sometimes my decisions went against the doctors' preferences. Regularly practicing *Healing Yoga* helped me to stay focused and calm, and to retain a sense of dignity. Similarly, regularly practicing *Healing Yoga* can help you manage the anxiety inherent in living with cancer.

The ongoing, deep fatigue of recovering from cancer treatments is very real and can be discouraging. Some days you may feel too tired to move. Unfortunately, inertia generates more inertia: without a manageable amount of exercise every day, you will probably feel even more exhausted. *Healing Yoga* is invigorating, adaptable

*See *Resources* (p. 115) for information about Cancer Lifeline.

for varying energy levels, and can be practiced in the privacy of your home.

Living with cancer, you may feel that your body has betrayed you. *Healing Yoga* can help you begin to feel at home in your body again. Through practicing *Healing Yoga*, you will begin to rebuild— and likely increase!—your physical strength, stamina, and flexibility through stretching, bending, twisting, and balancing movements combined with attention to a spacious, long breath. As a result of a regular *Healing Yoga* practice, you will once again experience yourself as resilient, powerful, and graceful.

Your *Healing Yoga* practice can also be a safe place for you to feel your emotions, even the "socially unacceptable" ones. For me, illness came with a range of feelings: fear, love, rage, peace, jealousy, gratitude, loneliness, intimacy, and boredom. Even though I had phenomenal support from my friends, family, and medical team, ultimately it was just me who had to bear being ill every day. Most of the time I focused on coping cheerfully, but in the privacy of my yoga practice I could let down my guard and, with compassion, witness my true emotions.

Finally, your *Healing Yoga* practice can help you tap into your sources of inner strength, courage, and fortitude. By using awareness and intention, you can fill your yoga practice with great personal meaning, so that your practice becomes an expression of your heart's deepest desires. You may come to experience your yoga practice as an offering or a prayer.

These are my wishes for you: May the quiet and reflective practices of *Healing Yoga* help you to come home to your body. May you—even as you adjust to living with cancer—live the most passionate, truthful, wonderful life possible, in intimate connection with your loved ones and with yourself.

Blessings to you—
Lisa Holtby

how to use this book

safety guidelines

If you are currently in active treatment for cancer or have lymphedema, please review this book with your oncologist or physician before trying the yoga poses. She/he can look at the photographs and put a check mark in the *Doctor's Okay* check box on each page to indicate if she/he feels the active poses in the chapters *Foundation, Ease, Strength,* and *Courage* are safe for you to practice at this time.

If you have bone metastases, open wounds, or if your platelet count is under 50,000, please do not practice the active poses in the chapters *Foundation*, *Ease*, *Strength*, and *Courage* without your physician's permission as they may be unsafe for you at this time.

It is safe to practice the chapters *Grace* and *Breath* at any stage of living with cancer.

practicing *healing yoga* during cancer treatments

If you are athletic: Practice *Healing Yoga* in combination with mild aerobic exercise, such as swimming or walking, as a bridge back to your normal workout.

If you already practice yoga regularly: Use *Healing Yoga* as a modified home practice until you feel ready to return to more vigorous classes.

If you are new to exercise: Try *Healing Yoga* as a satisfying and safe way to start!

clothing and yoga props

Wear comfortable clothes that you can move in easily. It is preferable to work with bare feet so that your feet do not slide. The *Resources* section p. 115) lists sources for yoga props. I strongly recommend using a yoga "sticky mat," but you may substitute a large towel instead. Throughout the book, I also mention use of a straight-backed chair and a yoga strap, block, blanket, and bolster. You may use substitutes for these items: sit on the edge of a firm bed rather than on a chair, use a bathrobe tie or towel instead of a yoga strap, substitute a rolled up towel for a yoga block, and use a firm blanket in place of a special yoga blanket, and firm couch cushion instead of a yoga bolster.

designing your yoga practice

Please begin each practice by reclining in Resting Pose (p. 19) for five to ten minutes and settling into a steady breath and into your heart, as described in the chapters *Grace* and *Breath*. Then, the poses and sequences are written to be practiced in succession so that you are thoroughly warmed up for the more challenging poses. For example:

If you wish to rest: Practice the chapters *Grace* and *Breath*.

If your balance feels unsteady, if you are fatigued, or if you are new to exercise: Begin your practice with the chapters *Grace* and *Breath*, then continue on to the chapter *Foundation*. Hold each pose in the *Foundation* sequence for a few long, relaxed breaths, then rest as needed before moving on to the next pose.

If you wish to rebuild your stamina and strength: Begin your practice with chapters *Grace*, *Breath*, and *Foundation*, then continue on to *Ease*. When you are able to practice these sequences comfortably, without feeling weary afterward, then add the sequence in *Strength*. Finally, as is appropriate for your energy level, add the sequence in *Courage*.

As you rebuild your strength, you may wish to hold each pose for several long, relaxed breaths. Or you may wish to hold each pose for only a few spacious, relaxed breaths, but practice each pose two or three times before moving on to the next. Try to flow slowly, like molasses, from one pose to the next. Another image is to move as if underwater, smoothly and gracefully.

working at an appropriate level

Similarly, I encourage you to practice *Healing Yoga* so that you do not experience any pain, but instead feel pleasantly challenged.

You are working at an appropriate level if:

- In each pose, you are able to maintain the steady, smooth breathing described in the chapter *Breath*, plus keep the muscles in your face and jaw relaxed.
- In each pose, any sensations of intensity stop as soon as you slowly come out of the pose. Sensations of intensity may include your muscles stretching, quivering, or feeling hot. It is also okay if the pose is just plain hard but does not cause you pain.

- After your yoga practice, you feel relaxed and refreshed, not exhausted or overwhelmed.

You are working too hard or need to modify the pose if:

- You notice that you are holding your breath or tightening up the muscles in your face and jaw. (Return to the deep, slow breathing described in the chapter *Breath*. On your exhales, invite your muscles to soften and relax.)
- You feel any sharp or stabbing sensations that do not go away when you slowly come out of the pose. (Skip the pose for today and seek the advice of an experienced yoga instructor.)
- After your yoga practice, you feel exhausted. (Please rest, and the next time you do yoga, hold the poses for shorter lengths of time and/or reduce the number of sequences that you practice.)
- You have lymphedema, and you feel tingling or swelling in your affected limb(s) after your yoga practice. Because physical activity increases the volume of lymphatic fluid in your body, it is important to monitor affected or at-risk areas for any changes. Similarly, so as not to increase swelling, add new yoga sequences—or any other new exercise programs—gradually. (Be sure to consult your physician to assess which poses are appropriate for you, always wear your protective cuff when practicing yoga, and skip any poses that place too much pressure on your affected limb[s.])

- You experience discomfort or intuitively sense that something is wrong in the areas where your body has been affected by cancer. (Try the modifications suggested or skip that pose for today. Then, please ask your physician if the pose is still safe for you, and if so, seek the advice of an experienced yoga instructor to help you modify the pose.)

finding a yoga class

In this book, I describe each of the forty yoga poses with text and one or two photographs. I offer options to modify or intensify most of the poses. However, the disadvantage of not being in a yoga class together is that I cannot help you to modify the poses to fit your needs.

While I hope that you practice *Healing Yoga* at home, I also highly recommend attending gentle yoga classes designed for people living with cancer so that you can benefit from the group camaraderie, personalized instruction, and the structure of having regularly scheduled classes.

Right now, yoga is very popular in the United States, but unlike earning a degree in medicine, there is not a standardized licensing program to pursue before beginning to teach yoga. Please use discernment when shopping for a yoga teacher as there is tremendous variation in the quality of instruction offered.

Hopefully your medical center offers complementary therapies for people with living with cancer such as yoga and meditation classes, art therapy, support groups, and so on. If not, look for gentle yoga classes offered at yoga studios in your area.* It is worth asking yoga teachers to describe and quantify their training and teaching experience. For instance, if an instructor says she/he has been teaching for a decade, it is useful to know if she/he has been teaching off and on for those ten years, perhaps only teaching one class a week, or if she/he has been teaching full-time.

Similarly, please know that being a "certified yoga teacher" can mean having attended a week-long teacher training program, or it can mean qualifying after years of rigorous training and practice in not just in the yoga poses, but also philosophy, meditation, anatomy, teaching skills, and therapeutics.

Besides being knowledgeable, good yoga teachers will also be friendly and welcoming, will ask you before class if you have any injuries or health concerns, and will walk around during class to give individualized feedback and adjustments. Ultimately, the most important criteria for choosing a yoga class is that you feel safe physically and emotionally.

Finally, by reviewing this book with your physician and having her/him circle "yes" or "no" in the *Doctor's Okay* icon on each page, you will know which poses to avoid or modify in yoga classes. Also, you can show this book to your instructor to help her/him understand how to modify their class plans to meet your needs. She/he will probably be glad to help.

---

*See *Resources* (p. 115) for information on finding yoga classes in your area.

CHAPTER 3

healing yoga and cancer treatments

Not only will practicing *Healing Yoga* increase your energy, strength, flexibility, and sense of well-being, but it can also help you to recover from some of the side effects of cancer treatments and the impact of living with cancer.

stress

In response to crises, your muscles tense up, ready to spring into action. Your whole body goes into a "fight or flight" adrenaline state. You experience sweaty palms, a dry mouth, and a racing heart. Your breathing becomes fast and shallow. Your vision focuses sharply. Digestion slows down, as do the processes of cellular repair and renewal. This is your body's intelligent way of coping with emergencies. However, being in a chronic state of high alert is detrimental to managing the ongoing stress of living with cancer. Chronically tight muscles also limit your movements and can spasm painfully. *Healing Yoga* invites your body to relax. This not only feels restful but also frees up energy to support your body's ability to heal itself.

surgery

Post-surgery, until you have your physician's okay to exercise freely, it is still beneficial to stretch your unaffected side. Because of how the nervous system works, stretching an area on one side of the body indirectly benefits the same area on the opposite side of the body. For example, if you've had surgery (or radiation therapy) on your right leg, gently stretching and strengthening your left leg will directly benefit the left side and indirectly benefit that same area on the right side of the body that is still healing from treatment. Using the modifications suggested, *Healing Yoga* shows you how to stretch and strengthen safely.

anesthesia

General anesthesia used during surgery can affect cilia's ability to function. Cilia are like tiny hairs that line the inside of your lungs. Their natural wave action helps to eliminate secretions. If this action is inhibited and secretions accumulate, the results can range from a decrease in the normal exchange of oxygen and carbon dioxide to pneumonia. *Healing Yoga's* conscious breathing practice softens cilia so that they can once again function properly and protect your lungs.

lymph nodes removed

If you have had lymph nodes removed, *Healing Yoga's* conscious breathing and movements are especially useful. Lymphatic fluid supports your health by picking up viruses and pathogens in your system and taking them to your lymph nodes, clustered throughout your body, to be cleaned away. So, for instance, when you get a cut or sunburn, your body responds by sending more lymphatic fluid to the affected area to help it heal. But, if you've had lymph nodes removed, your body may be unable to handle the extra flow of lymph. The extra lymphatic fluid stays in the affected area, causing swelling, or lymphedema. Lymphedema also inhibits lymphatic fluid's gaseous exchange and cleansing functions, which, as a result, increase the risks of infection, changes in skin color and texture, and increased scar tissue within the deeper tissues. Manual lymph drainage massage helps to move lymph in the absence of lymph nodes. **Healing Yoga is not a replacement for this specialized massage**, but can help increase the overall circulation of lymph in your body.

Another side effect of having lymph nodes removed is that if lymphatic fluid is not circulating properly, it cannot lubricate your layers of muscle and fascia. As a result, you feel stiff. Lymphatic fluid bathes the tissues of the body so that they glide easily on top of one another. As the lymphatic system has no pumping mechanism, it is your physical movements that propel lymphatic fluid throughout your body. *Healing Yoga* massages lymphatic fluid through your tissues so that your movements are free and comfortable. Even the spacious, slow breathing described in the chapter *Breath* will help move lymph through your body.

scar tissue from radiation therapy and surgery

For the first year following radiation therapy or surgery, it is particularly important to regularly stretch around the affected area to prevent the resulting scar tissues from permanently limiting your range of motion. Radiation therapy uses high-dose x-ray beams to kill or damage cancer cells that grow and divide more rapidly than normal cells. Radiation therapy can also injure or kill normal cells in the area being treated, causing possible treatment side effects. One possible side effect of radiation therapy is like an internal (and sometimes external) burn injury that will scar, Radiation therapy can also burn blood vessels, which decreases circulation. Most normal cells damaged by radiation therapy eventually recover from the effects of the treatment, but some die and form a scar tissue called "diffuse fibrosis."

The scar tissue, or "incisional adhesions," that result from surgery are of a more localized nature. They may also limit joint mobility. For example, if you've had a mastectomy, regularly stretching your chest, shoulder, and arm helps you maintain or regain mobility in your shoulder joint and chest wall. The collagen strands that comprise normal tissue are shaped like long rubber bands lying side by side. But in scar tissue, collagen strands lie in a jumble, like a haystack. *Healing Yoga* helps realign the scar tissue's collagen strands again so that the scar tissue sets in a way that supports your ongoing ease of movement.

CHAPTER 4

grace

Wherever you are on your journey with cancer, you can safely practice the sequences in chapters *Grace* and *Breath*. These sequences cultivate mental and physical relaxation, and are the starting point for the rest of your yoga practice.

When I was new to yoga, I focused on the joyous physicality of the practice. My intent was to build the strength, flexibility, and stamina needed to achieve certain poses and to keep up in advanced classes. While satisfying and empowering, ultimately this way of practicing yoga lacked heart and meaning for me. These days, I still revel in the physical practice, but I also honor and express my heartfelt truths and desires, my true self, on my yoga mat. Practicing yoga now feels holy and filled with grace.

How you define the source of grace is entirely personal. Over the years, I have taught yoga to people of many diverse faiths, to people who define themselves as nonreligious spiritual seekers, and to atheists. The nondenominational practices of yoga are available to people of all wisdom traditions, whether you understand the source of grace to be God, the Divine, Mother Mary, Mother Nature, Buddha Nature, Shiva and Shakti, the best of the human spirit, or the power of love.

Here is my personal experience of opening to grace in my yoga practice. I begin by sitting quietly and comfortably for five minutes or so, with eyes closed, and settle into the spacious, steady breathing detailed in the chapter *Breath*. I don't try to push thoughts away, nor do I try to "think positively." Rather, my mind begins to quiet through the process of resting my awareness on each breath and watching its effect on my body. Focusing on my body and breath during yoga feels, to me, like being completely engrossed in an exciting project or a gripping book. Because my own little world becomes so interesting, I'm only tangentially aware of sounds around me and other people in the room.

As I sit quietly, I take note of how I truly feel, both physically and emotionally. While the truth is not always pretty, I try not to ignore or deny my feelings. For instance, I may begin my yoga practice alternately concerned about a friend's health, angry about an argument I just had, and thinking about an upcoming deadline. Rather than pushing those thoughts away or judging myself for them, I try to be a compassionate witness for whatever is true. Especially when times are hard, I try to be as kind to myself as I am to my sweet toddler when he bumps his head and cries.

Then I move into a slow, steady flow of yoga poses, such as the sequences detailed in chapters *Foundation*, *Ease*, *Strength*, and *Courage*. I pay attention to my alignment, observe my breath—and occasionally think about how mad I am and also that I need to pick up milk and bananas. While the constant chatter of my thoughts, of worries and plans and memories, may still be there, it's as if the volume keeps going down on that part of my mind. Gradually, most of my awareness becomes quiet and expansive. Beneath the chatter of my thoughts lie deeper truths. From that place of truthfulness, I then make a dedication for my practice.

What often happens is that a dedication just bubbles up, usually toward the beginning of my practice as I am sitting quietly or warming up in the first few poses. For me, this unveiling comes as a result of bringing my awareness into the present moment, which I do by resting my attention on how the sensations of my breath and body change in response to each slow inhale and exhale.

For instance, if what bubbles up is sadness and fear for my friend who is ill, then I dedicate my practice to her. I visualize her face, or imagine holding her hands in mine. I might imagine moving strongly for her at a time when she cannot. I might envision surrounding her with love, like wrapping a soft quilt around her shoulders. I might embody peaceful images, as if I could move as easily as a fish in calm waters, or stand as tranquil and still as a mountain. Sometimes words or phrases float through my mind, like "mercy," or "this too shall pass," or "peace be with you."

If what bubbles up are strong feelings of anger, I may choose to dedicate my practice to cultivating inner strength and courage. I might channel that fiery energy into stoking up my practice. I may move energetically, challenge myself by holding poses for few breaths longer than usual, and visualize myself as a warrior standing tall and proud. Conversely, I may choose to dedicate my practice to clarity, slowing down my movements so that I have time to thoughtfully explore each pose and to listen for inner wisdom.

Even on very bad days, often what bubbles up is gratitude—or a deep yearning to dwell in gratitude—and I dedicate my practice accordingly. When I take my arms out to the side in a pose, I might imagine that I'm opening my arms wide into an embrace. When I come into a spinal twist, I may visualize turning toward my loved ones. While practicing, I might suddenly realize that I owe my husband an apology, or that I have multitasked so efficiently that I haven't truly connected with my little boy that day. Images come to me, like of my son hippity-hopping around our home, singing little songs to himself, or the wonderful smell of my husband's neck, or how lovely this pose feels. Sometimes I feel great joy well up inside me, like my heart could burst with gladness.

During hard times when there's no joy or gladness to be found, even experiencing glimmers of peace or hope during my yoga practice have helped to sustain me.

There are rich results to dedicating my practice. Even after more than a decade of doing yoga, I am always surprised when, focusing on my breath and the details of whatever pose I am in, I receive a flash of understanding, or an extraordinary inspiration, or a jaw-dropping realization. Also, my intentions for my practice spill over into the rest of my day. Seemingly without effort or thought, I act in ways congruent with my intentions. I find the strength to do hard things. I gain perspective, so that small problems don't bother me as much. I feel happy. I have more patience. Or, I become extremely impatient with situations that I've realized drain me and that I need to end with integrity.

Practicing yoga with intention helps me to act with clarity, truthfulness, and kindness in my daily life. I attribute the results of my yoga practice as gifts of grace.

Certainly not every practice is life-changing for me. Most of the time after yoga I just feel pleasantly refreshed. But over time, yoga has been both transformational and an oasis of peace as I have opened myself to grace.

And so, as you practice the breathing and yoga poses in this book, I invite you to open yourself to grace. I invite you to bring all of your emotions and thoughts to your yoga practice, even if what you feel is overwhelming fear, or rage at your cancer, or grief that you have lost your hair or a part of your body. Fully experiencing what is true for you in the moment will give rise to your heartfelt dedication for your practice, so that your yoga practice embodies and reflects your heart's fierce desires.

breath

I have found that if I do not settle myself into a smooth, full, and spacious breath before and during my practice, then I experience yoga as dull. Time passes slowly. By contrast, when I bring my attention to my breath and invite it to lengthen and deepen, then my practice feels meditative. I become fascinated by exquisite subtleties of sensation. I experience yoga as uplifting. Indeed, the name of the breathing practice in Sanskrit is *ujjayi*, or "victorious uprising." In the yoga poses, I feel my body respond to my breath, so that I stabilize on each inhale and expand radiantly on each exhale. For me, a steady *ujjayi* breath feels like coming home.

full belly breathing

Let's begin! You can learn the breathing practices right now, as you are reading along. (Or you may wish to have someone read aloud to you.) Please sit comfortably upright in bed, on a chair, or on the floor. If you need to lie down, that's fine. If you can, breathe in and out through your nose with your lips gently closed. Rest your right hand on your belly and your left hand on your chest (photo 1). As you breathe, do you feel more movement happening underneath your right hand resting on your belly, or underneath your left hand resting on your chest?

Here's an experiment: Try exaggerating breathing high into your chest so that you feel very little movement in your belly. Just for fun, scowl. Clench your jaw. Tighten your belly. Is your breath shallow as a result? When your breath is high in your chest and short, your heart rate increases and your nervous system responds by going into a "fight or flight" adrenaline response, especially if the muscles in your face and belly are also tense. If breathing this way feels normal to you, then practicing full belly breathing will be especially helpful.

Now, relax your face, jaw, shoulders, and belly. Soften your gaze. Imagine breathing way down deep into the very bottom of your lungs. Slow down your breath, so that every inhale and exhale feels full and complete. Do you experience a sense of relief when your body and breath begin to relax? And do you notice more expansion of your belly into your right hand? Your heart rate has probably slowed down, and your deep, smooth breathing signals your nervous system to calm down as well. This is the full belly breath that you will sustain throughout your yoga practice. Please rest your hands comfortably in your lap, close your eyes, and enjoy breathing for a few minutes.

When you feel ready to continue, let's look at how full belly breathing works. When your breath is deep and spacious, you will feel expansion and release in your belly. To clarify, you're not using your surface abdominal muscles to push your belly outward into your hand. Rather, your torso is divided into two sections—like upstairs and downstairs apartments—by your diaphragm muscle, a powerful sheath of muscle that looks something like an open parachute nestled inside of your ribcage. In the "upstairs apartment" are your lungs and heart. Below your diaphragm muscle, in the "downstairs apartment," are your digestive and reproductive organs, very tightly packed in. When you inhale deeply, to make room for your lungs to expand magnificently, your diaphragm muscle presses down against your digestive organs. When those organs are momentarily compressed, they press outward, and so you feel your belly expanding. When you exhale and your lungs deflate, then your diaphragm muscle floats back up in the direction of your heart and your belly settles back in the direction of your spine. It's as if your diaphragm muscle is a

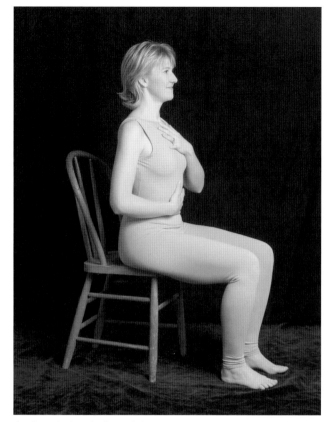

| Breathe into belly and chest

trampoline upon which your lungs are jumping up and down in slow motion. The play between your diaphragm and lungs also massages your heart. So full belly breathing strengthens your respiratory, lymphatic and circulatory systems, nourishes the exchange of oxygen at a cellular level, and soothes your nervous system.

Now let's bring even greater fullness to your breath. Please rest your hands on the back of your ribcage (photo 2). When you inhale, imagine sending your breath to the back side of your body. As a result, you may feel the back of your ribcage

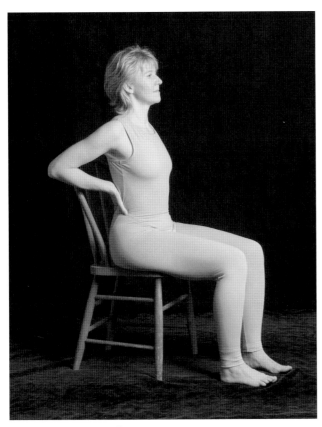

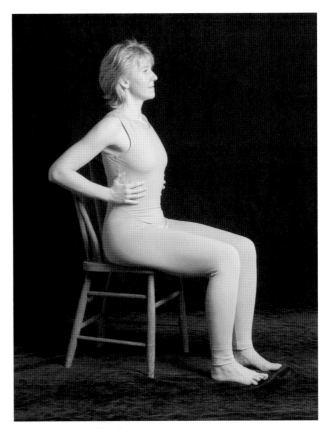

2   Breathe into back ribs

3   Breathe into side ribs

expand and release with your breath. You may notice an undulation along your spine, or a slight widening and then release of your shoulder blades on your back. Again, these subtle movements are a result of breathing deeply and not something you need to make happen through muscular effort.

As you direct your breath into the back of your body, you may notice more sensation in your back body as well. Imagine the front of your body as passive, relaxed. Let your face soften. Here's another experiment: try to sense the parameters of your back body. For instance, can you feel where

the very top of your head is? How wide your shoulders are? The touch of your clothes against your back? Air currents against your bare skin?

Now rest your hands on the left and right sides of your ribcage (photo 3). Breathe into your hands, so that when you inhale, the expansion of your lungs widens your ribcage laterally. When you exhale, the sides of your ribcage float back toward the midline of your body, away from your hands. Not only do your lungs expand laterally, out into your hands, but also medially, toward the midline of your body. On your inhales, envision the inner aspects of your lungs expanding toward one another underneath your breastbone.

Please rest your hands comfortably in your lap. As you bring more attention to the subtleties of your breath, have any muscles in your face, jaw, or shoulders clenched with the effort of noticing? Invite those muscles to relax.

Imagine inhaling rich, oxygenated air all the way deep into the bottom of your lungs so that your lungs feel wide. Continue inhaling up into what feels like the middle of your lungs, then into the top of your lungs underneath your collarbones. On your exhales, easily and slowly release your breath. A slightly extended exhalation, perhaps two or three seconds longer than your inhalation, is an especially calming practice.

Let's put all of this together. Imagine, now, breathing into the whole circumference of your ribcage—into the back of your ribcage, the sides, the front, way down deep into the bottom of your lungs, and all the way to the top of your lungs underneath your collarbones. Cultivate just the right balance of effort and ease so that your breath feels nourishing, but without trying so hard that your throat tightens up or you feel anxious. It's a fine line between directing your breath and forcing your breath. If you observe that you are pushing for a particular result, say, holding your breath to make it longer, then give up the struggle and simply breathe.

During full belly breathing, you may feel your whole body rocking ever so slightly in response to each inhale and exhale, like you are bodysurfing over the gentle waves of your breath.

Not only is full belly breathing deep, but it is also long and slow. You might notice a short pause at the top of your inhale, just before the exhalation begins of its own accord. There may be long or short pauses at the end of your exhale, just before the inhalation arises of its own accord. Rest quietly in the stillness between breaths.

ujjayi breathing

Here is a final distinction that transforms your full belly breathing into the "victorious uprising" of *ujjayi* breathing. When you breathe long and slow, in and out of your nose, your breath will create a little hissing sound at the back of your throat. (This is different than creating a humming sound with your vocal cords.) For me, the hiss of my breath sounds like ocean waves heard from a distance. By hollowing the back of your throat slightly, you will both lengthen your breath and amplify the *ujjayi* sound. To find this shape in your mouth and throat, pretend you are fogging a mirror with your breath, or breathing on your sunglasses before polishing them. Your exhales will make a little "hhhaaaa" sound. The *ujjayi* breath is the very same feeling and action, just with your lips lightly closed and jaw relaxed. Similarly, try whispering. When you whisper, you create the same feeling and action in your mouth and throat as when you practice *ujjayi* breathing, again, just with your lips lightly closed and jaw relaxed.

When *ujjayi* breathing feels restful and perhaps meditative, please continue on to Resting Pose.

resting pose

I invite you to begin and end your yoga practices with Resting Pose. Please lie on your back on a firm bed or on a yoga mat on the floor. Use layers of evenly folded blankets underneath you if you need extra padding. Position your body so that your head is in line with your pelvis and your arms and legs are equal distances away from the midline of your body. Turn your palms up to face the sky. As your legs relax, they will turn out slightly, away from the midline of your body. Notice if your chin is level with your forehead. If your chin points up toward the sky, the back of your neck is probably shortening, so place a neatly folded blanket underneath your head to lengthen the back of your neck. If your lower back feels uncomfortable, try elevating your lower legs on a firm bolster or smoothly folded blankets (photo 4). If needed, cover yourself with extra blankets to stay warm.

For the extra deluxe version of Resting Pose, use an eye-pillow.[*] These are often made of silk

[*] See *Resources* (p. 115) for information on ordering yoga props.

and filled with fragrant flaxseed and lavender, and can be warmed in a microwave. The light pressure and warmth of the pillow against your eyes helps the muscles of your face to relax and your mind to quiet down.

Settle into your *ujjayi* breath. With your inhalations, notice how your body gently expands. With your exhalations, notice how your body softens. Resting Pose is a form of conscious relaxation, so your mind stays alert while your body relaxes deeply. However, if you drift off to sleep, you probably need the rest, so enjoy a little nap!

Breath by breath, surrender the weight of your body into the earth. Perhaps imagine being cradled by a loving mother, or held in the arms of your god. When your mind wanders, notice your thoughts, then gently bring your awareness back to the expansion of this inhalation, the release of this exhalation, the truth of this present moment. Rest in the stillness between your breaths.

If your mind is jumping around like drunken monkeys, as the Buddhists say, is it possible to simply witness your thoughts for a few minutes? To watch your thoughts the way you would watch storm clouds scudding by in the sky? It helps me to realize that my thoughts are not necessarily accurate reflections of reality. "Hmmm, here I go making up disaster scenarios again: this is not reality." "I'm arguing with someone in my head again: this is not reality." Or you may simply label the type of thoughts

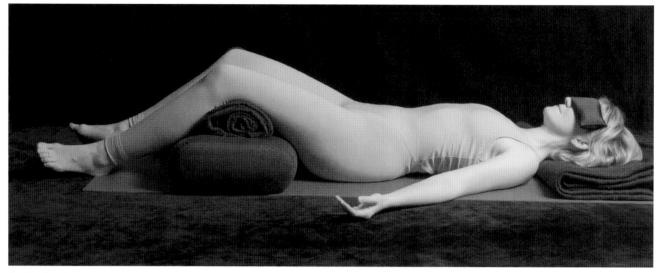

4   Resting Pose

and emotions you are having as an observer ("fear . . . anger . . . planning . . . remembering") rather than getting caught up in the drama of your story. Observing your thoughts is rather like watching a train thunder past you and noting the different kinds of cars on it ("engine . . . passenger car . . . box car . . . caboose") instead of leaping onto the train itself. When I watch my thoughts as a compassionate witness, I learn how my mind habitually functions. When I know what my reflexive reactions are, then I begin to have more choice as to how I think, act, and perceive reality.

After five to ten minutes in Resting Pose, or when you feel ready, deepen your breath again. Take your time coming back up to sitting. You might like to roll onto your side and rest there for a few breaths. Then, using your hands on the floor or bed, press up to sitting again.

Take note of how you feel after simply breathing with intention for a few minutes. You may be breathing easier. You may feel focused and also relaxed. This may be a good time to consciously open to grace. Please notice, with compassion, the truth of this present moment. How do you feel, physically, emotionally, and mentally? From what is true for you, perhaps you would like to dedicate your practice on behalf of yourself or someone else. What are your heart's desires right now? For healing? Peace? Mercy? Courage? You may come to experience each breath and gesture in your yoga practice as an embodiment and expression of your deepest longings for transformation.

As you are ready, please continue on to the next chapter, *Foundation*.

foundation

What differentiates a yoga practice from simply exercising is the integration—and steady awareness—of your heart's intention, your breath, and your movements. So before trying this first sequence of active poses, please settle into your *ujjayi* breath and into your heart while reclining in Resting Pose, as described in the previous chapters *Grace* and *Breath*.

Foundation is complete practice by itself if you feel fatigued or your balance feels unsteady, or you are new to exercise. Please remember to practice the poses in this chapter sequentially, skipping any poses or variations that feel unsafe or painful.

If you feel energized, *Foundation* is great warm-up for the following three chapters. Please slowly work through the *Foundation* sequence before moving on to *Ease* or *Strength* and *Courage*.

While the poses in this chapter are simple, they are also rich in detail. You will learn anatomical terms and principles of alignment, practice the basic movements of *Healing Yoga* (lengthening, arching, rounding, folding, and twisting), and explore the balance in each pose between strength and expansion.

You will practice this sequence of ten poses while seated in a straight-backed chair.

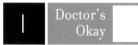

SEATED MOUNTAIN
Modified Tadasana

Seated Mountain establishes a strong foundation from which to lengthen and expand. Sit tall and relaxed in Mountain, with great dignity. Try Mountain as you drive, or work at your desk, or talk with your medical team.

benefits
Lengthens spine, opens chest, relaxes shoulders

how to set up
Sit upright in a straight-backed chair. Settle your feet flat on the ground, parallel to one another and hips' width apart. Rest your hands at your **hip creases.** To create a gentle concavity or arch in your lower back, lean your torso forward about twelve inches as you float your collarbones upward, as if they were wings. Tilt the front of your **pelvis** forward (photo 5). As a result, you'll feel your lower back arch. (To check, take your fingers along your spine at your lower back. When your lower back is arched, the bumpy line of your spine recedes deep into your body instead of poking out into your hand.)

Keep the slight arch in your lower back, sit upright once again, with your heart lifted and proud. Allow your shoulder blades to rest on your back. Lengthen the back of your pelvis—ending in your **tailbone**—down toward the earth, like sending down roots. Tip the front of your pelvis—your **pubic bone***—up toward the sky. You will feel your abdominal muscles tone as a result. Rest your hands on your thighs, palms down (photo 6).

Energize your feet: lift and widen your toes. Sense the four "corners" on the soles of your feet: mound of your big toe, inner heel, outer heel, mound of your little toe. Press the **four corners of your feet*** down.

Gently slide your head straight back so that your ears line up over your shoulders and hips—for most of us, that's only a movement of an inch or so. Slightly lengthen up through the back of your head. The back of your neck will strengthen subtly.

on your inhalations
Notice the expansion of your ribcage as you draw in a spacious breath. Relax your face, eyes, and jaw.

on your exhalations
Lightly press down through your lower legs and feet into the ground, and your **sit bones*** into the chair seat. Lengthen upward through your spine. Like a gentle hug, firm your belly ever so slightly back toward your spine. Even as you are strengthening and lengthening, relax your shoulders. Notice how soft and tactile your skin is. Soften the muscles around your eyes. For a few minutes, sit quietly, solid and powerful as a mountain. Then continue on to Seated Cat.

*See *Anatomy Notes* (p. 109) for descriptions of these terms.

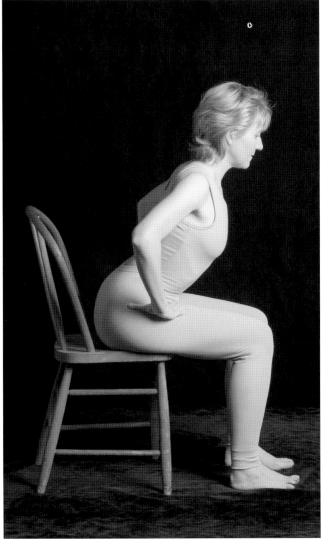

5 Seated Mountain preparation

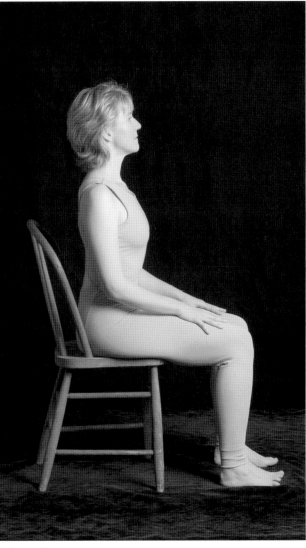

6 Seated Mountain

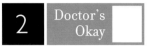

2 Doctor's Okay

SEATED CAT
Modified Bidalasana

To me, this pose feels private, contemplative. Curling into yourself, you can hear and feel your breath more clearly, and draw into your own quiet wisdom.

benefits
Stretches upper and middle back

how to set up
Sit in Mountain. Interlace your fingers and turn your palms forward, away from your chest. Round your spine back as you stretch your arms forward.

on your inhalations
Relax your face. Notice how your shoulder blades widen on your back, like great wings spreading open.

on your exhalations
Hollow your belly and chest back toward your spine. Press your palms further forward as you round your spine further back, lithe and graceful as a cat (photo 7).

to finish
Release your hands and rest in Mountain. When you feel ready, continue on to Seated Twist.

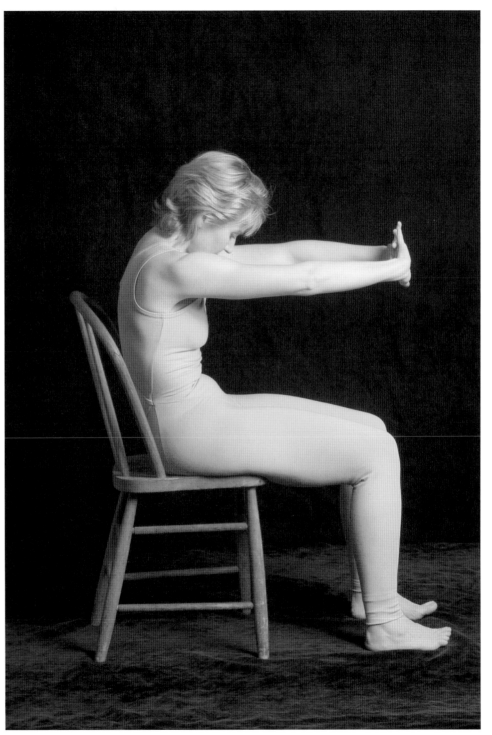

7   Seated Cat

SEATED TWIST
Modified Bharadvajasana

Whereas Cat is a turning in toward oneself, I experience spinal twists as a turning toward others. Imagine turning to someone who adores you, and basking in his or her love for you, like standing in sunlight.

benefits
Releases back tension, lengthens spine

how to set up
Sit in Mountain. Press your feet down into the earth. Slowly turn your upper body to the right, into a spinal twist. Keep your head directly over your pelvis rather than leaning your torso to the right. Press both sit bones down into the chair seat.

on your inhalations
Expand your ribcage with your breath. Relax your shoulders, face, and jaw. Your spacious inhales will momentarily unwind the twist just a little in your torso.

on your exhalations
Deepen the twist. Initiate this deeper twist from the power of your back body. Imagine your spine like a tall, strong pole, and your outer body—your belly, rib cage, chest, neck and head—wrapping around the pole like bright ribbons around a maypole.

to intensify
Use your hands as leverage on the chair or on your right leg to bring you deeper into the twist (photo 8). As you turn to the right, your left leg and hip will tend to slide forward. To level your hips again, slide your left thigh back, and draw the top of your thighbone more deeply into its hip socket. At the same time, press down through your right leg and foot.

to finish
Slowly unwind. Rest in center for a few long breaths. When you feel ready, try the pose on the second side, then continue on to Seated Wings.

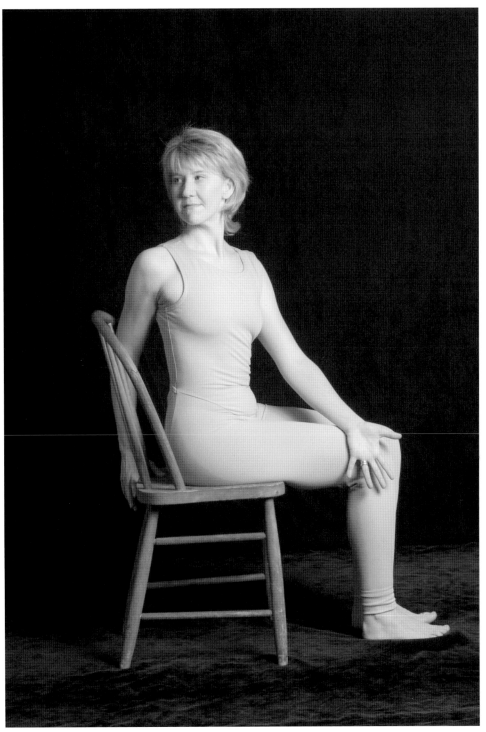

8   Seated Twist

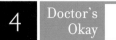

SEATED WINGS

How you hold your body affects your emotional state. If you sit slumped over, with shoulders rounded and head hanging, you probably will start to feel dejected. By contrast, sitting in Wings increases your energy. From the strong foundation of sitting in Mountain, you then rise up through your spine and widen your arms, like a powerful bird spreading its wings.

benefits
Strengthens upper back, opens chest

how to set up
Sit in Mountain. Lightly shrug your shoulders up and strongly roll the **head of your arm bones*** back. Let your shoulder blades press onto your back, as if they were two strong, friendly hands lifting up your heart. With the head of your arm bones still rolled back, extend your arms out to the sides at right angles, elbows at shoulder height and forearms up toward the sky, rather like the shape of a saguaro cactus. Reach your elbows and upper arms forward as you press your lower arms and hands back, as if you want to point at something with your elbows. As a result, your chest will lift and you will feel strong in your upper back, even

as the top of your shoulders stay wide and relaxed (photo 9).

on your inhalations
Soften your face and jaw. Relax the muscles around your eyes. If your chin juts forward, slide your head straight back an inch or so. Slightly lengthen up through the back of your head. The back of your neck will strengthen subtly.

on your exhalations
So that you don't overarch your lower back, lengthen your tailbone down toward the earth. Like a gentle hug, firm your belly toward your spine.

to intensify
Reach out from the center of your chest and back to extend your arms out wide, all the way through your fingertips. Press your arms straight back, as if you were soaring high in the sky (photo 10).

to finish
Release your arms and rest your hands easily in your lap. When you feel ready, continue on to Seated Half Moon.

---

* See *Anatomy Notes* (p. 109) for a description of this term.

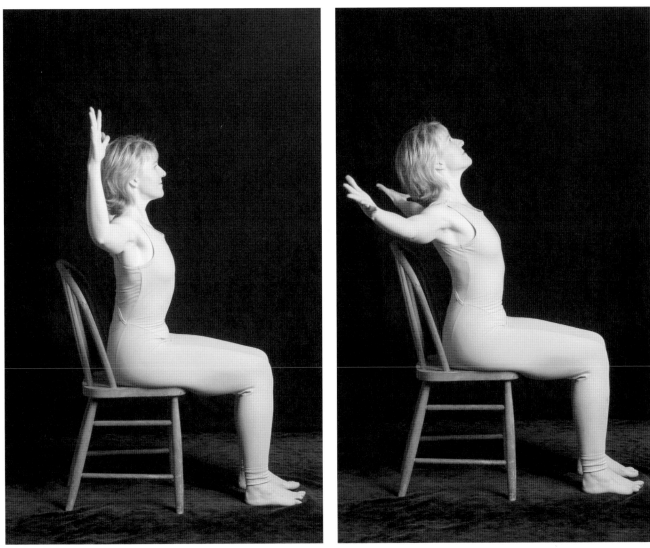

9   Seated Wings modified

10 Seated Wings intensified

SEATED HALF MOON
Modified Ardha Chandrasana

Seated Half Moon is an exploration of the paradox inherent in all yoga poses: finding the balance between stability and lightness, roots and wings.

benefits
Stretches muscles on the sides of your torso, facilitates deeper breathing

how to set up
Sit in Mountain. Lightly shrug your shoulders up, strongly roll the head of your arm bones back. Keep your shoulder blades comfortably wide and draw them magnetically onto your back. Press both sitbones into the chair seat and feet into the ground. Slowly lengthen your torso up and over to the right into a side bend. Rest your left hand on the left side of your ribcage and right hand on the chair legs or rungs. Rather than letting your upper body slump to the right, lengthen your torso up and over, as if reaching over a huge ball balanced at the right side of your waist (photo 11).

on your inhalations
Imagine inhaling bright, luminous energy. Soften your face and jaw.

on your exhalations
With each exhale, imagine sending that luminous energy out through your arms, down through your legs and sit bones, and all the way along your spine up to the top of your head. Envision expanding outward.

to intensify
Re-commit to a strong foundation: press your sit bones and feet down, roll the head of your arm bones back, and firm your shoulder blades onto your back. Now stretch your left arm way out to the left, palm up. Slowly draw a big arc with your arm. Reach high overhead and over to the right, like the shape of a crescent moon, free and light (photo 12).

to finish
Float your left arm down and bring your torso back up to center. Rest for a few breaths. Notice how the left side of your torso feels. Does your left lung feel more spacious and open than your right lung? When you feel ready, try the pose on the second side, then continue on to Seated Cobra.

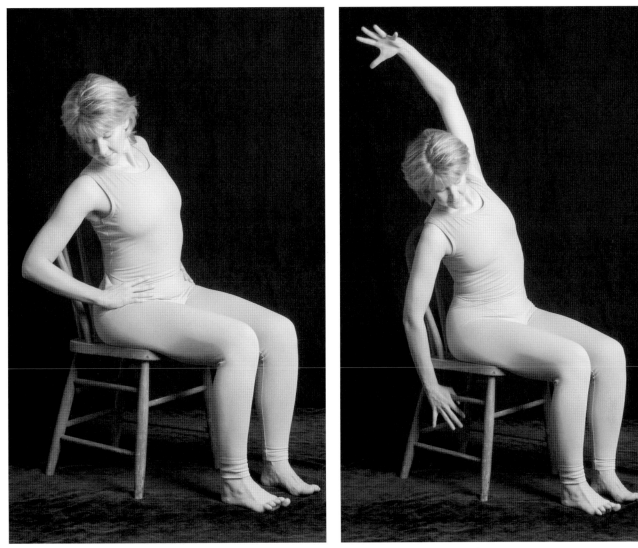

11 Seated Half Moon modified

12 Seated Half Moon intensified

SEATED COBRA
Modified Bhujangasana

Backbends require the courage to drop back into the unknown and unseen. In this pose, you begin with the solidity of sitting in Mountain. You may wish to envision your friends, family, and medical team all standing behind you, supporting you in this backbend, as you move courageously into the unknown.

benefits
Opens chest, strengthens back

how to set up
Sit in Mountain. Lightly shrug your shoulders up, strongly roll the head of your arm bones back. Keep your shoulder blades comfortably wide and press your shoulder blades onto your back. Interlace your hands behind your head with your elbows wide.

on your inhalations
Feel the expansion of your ribcage with your breath. Relax your face and jaw.

on your exhalations
Lift your chest so that your heart shines out and your collarbones float up and widen. Cascade back into a deeper arch, as if you could go up and over the chair back. Support the weight of your head in your hands. So that you don't overarch your lower back, firm your belly back toward your spine and lengthen your tailbone down toward the earth (photo 13).

to intensify
Notice the difference between initiating the backbend only from the *front* of your chest versus the back and front of your torso.

In my experience, when I lift my heart primarily by jamming my chest forward and up, my lower back tightens up and the movement feels aggressive, full of false bravado, and unsustainable.

Instead, lift your heart from the power of your upper back, as if friendly hands are supporting you. At the same time, imagine your heart easily floating up, soft and receptive, to receive that support.

to finish
Release your arms and rest your hands comfortably in your lap. When you feel ready, continue on to Seated Warrior I.

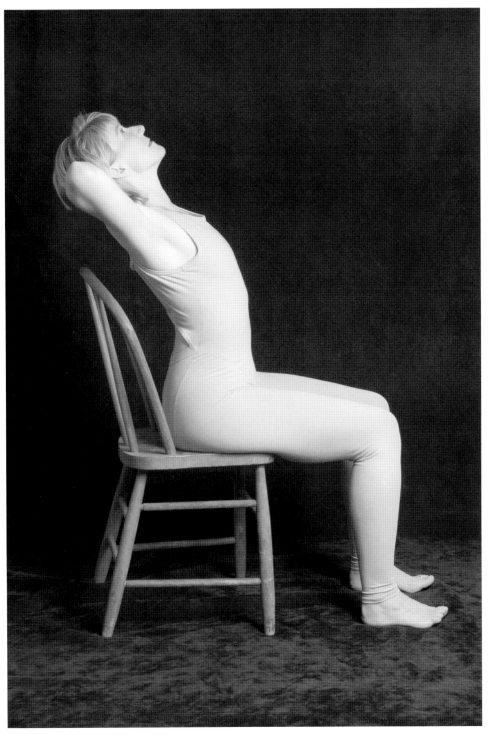

13 Seated Cobra

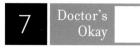
SEATED WARRIOR I
Modified Virabhadrasana I

In Seated Warrior I, you draw inward, into your own strength and resolve, and then expand outward, like a warrior courageously leaping into battle.

benefits
Stretches hips and legs, lengthens spine

how to set up
Sit sideways on the chair so that the right side of your body and right leg almost touch the chair back. Keep a long spine, as in Mountain, and step your left leg back, foot flexed, and balls of your toes on the ground. Rest your hands on the chair seat and back (photo 14).

on your inhalations
Draw your right thigh strongly *back* to nestle the top of your thigh bone deeper into its hip joint, and your left thigh strongly *forward* to settle it deeper into its hip joint. Lengthen your tailbone down toward the earth and your pubic bone up toward the sky. These movements are subtle, but the results are powerful: notice how your hip bones line up evenly across and your pelvis feels strong and compact.

on your exhalations
Keep your legs strongly drawn into their hip joints and also extend your legs longer, like a runner in midstride. Extend your right knee forward. Reach your left heel back toward the wall behind you. Lift your left inner thigh up toward the sky.

to intensify
Lightly shrug your shoulders up, strongly roll the head of your arm bones back, and press your shoulder blades onto your back. Boldly sweep your arms forward and overhead in a big arc, palms facing one another. On your exhalations, lift up your heart and reach your arms further back behind you (photo 15).

to finish
Slowly release your arms down. Rest sitting with your back against the chair back. When you feel ready, try the pose on the second side, then continue on to Seated Revolved Side Angle.

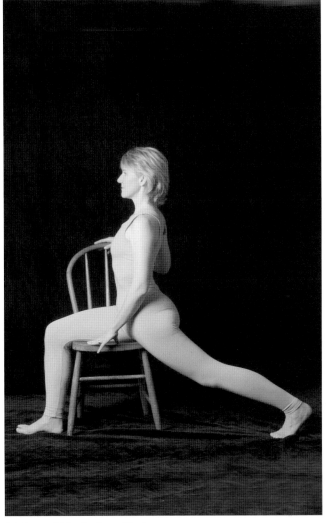

14 Seated Warrior I modified

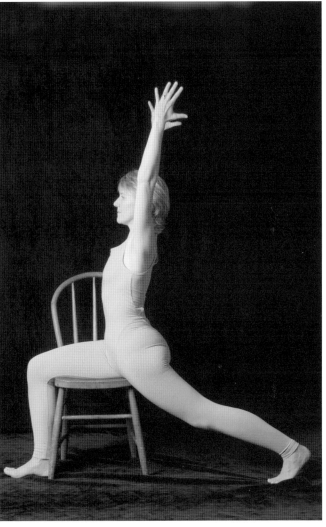

15 Seated Warrior I intensified

SEATED REVOLVED SIDE ANGLE

Modified Parivritta Parsvakonasana

Seated Revolved Side Angle embodies the stability of Seated Mountain, the individual effort of Seated Warrior I, the turning toward community support of Seated Twist, and the open-hearted expansion of Wings.

benefits

Stretches hips and legs, releases back tension, lengthens spine

how to set up

Set up in Warrior I: sit sideways in the chair so the right side of your body and right leg face the chair back, and reach your left leg back. As in Warrior I, stabilize your pelvis and energize your legs. Now, as in Seated Twist, slowly turn your upper body to the right, into a spinal twist. Use your hands on the chair back to help you deepen into the twist (photo 16).

on your inhalations

Deepen your roots: draw your thigh bones strongly into their hip joints, lengthen your tailbone down toward the earth, and tilt your pubic bone up toward the sky.

on your exhalations

Spread your wings: spiral further upward and to the right into a delicious spinal twist. If you wish, extend your arms outward from your heart. Reach out with wide arms to embrace all the paradoxes of being human: love and loss, vulnerability and strength, fear and grace (photo 17).

to finish

Slowly unwind out of the twist and release your arms down. Rest sitting with your back against the chair back. When you feel ready, try the pose on the second side, then continue on to Seated Half Lotus.

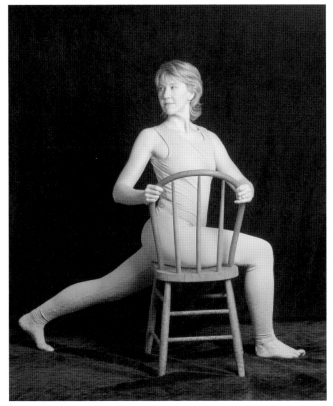

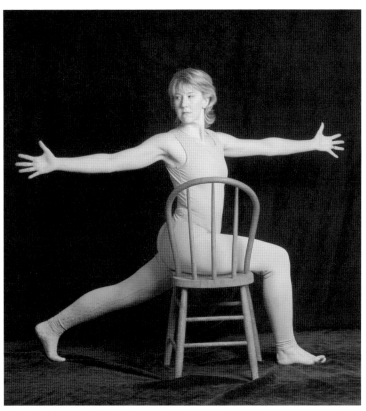

16 Seated Revolved Side Angle modified

17 Seated Revolved Side Angle intensified

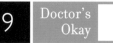
SEATED HALF LOTUS PREPARATION
Modified Ardha Padmasana

This pose requires an attitude of fierce commitment in order to stay with the intensity of the stretch in your hips. Paradoxically, you also bow forward. To me, the bow feels like a gesture of acceptance.

benefits
Stretches outer hips and buttocks

how to set up
Sit in Mountain. Cross your right ankle over your left thigh, just above your left knee. From Mountain, do you remember the actions to engage the muscles in your feet and lower legs? Widen and lengthen your toes, flex both feet so that you draw your toes back toward your shins. Sense the four "corners" on the soles of your feet: mound of your big toe, inner heel, outer heel, and mound of your little toe. Pressing out through these four points will intensify the stretch in your right hip.

Lightly shrug your shoulders up, strongly roll the head of your arm bones back, and press your shoulder blades onto your back. Take your hands to your hip creases. With your heart lifted and spine long, begin to fold forward, toward resting your chest and belly onto your legs (photo 18).

on your inhalations
Seek a balance between intensity and softness. Where do you *not* need to work hard? For instance, do you need to grit your teeth or hunch your shoulders in order to stretch your outer hip?

on your exhalations
Keep your spine long, heart lifted, and the head of your arm bones rolled back. Fold more deeply forward from your hip creases. To visualize how to fold at your hip creases, imagine your pelvis like a bowl filled with water. Tip the bowl—the front of your pelvis—forward to pour the water down into the earth.

to finish
Float your torso back upright again and step your right foot to the ground. Do the left and right sides of your pelvis feel different? You may notice that your right hip and leg feel more relaxed and heavy than your left hip and leg. When you feel ready, try the pose on the second side, then continue on to Seated Neck Stretch.

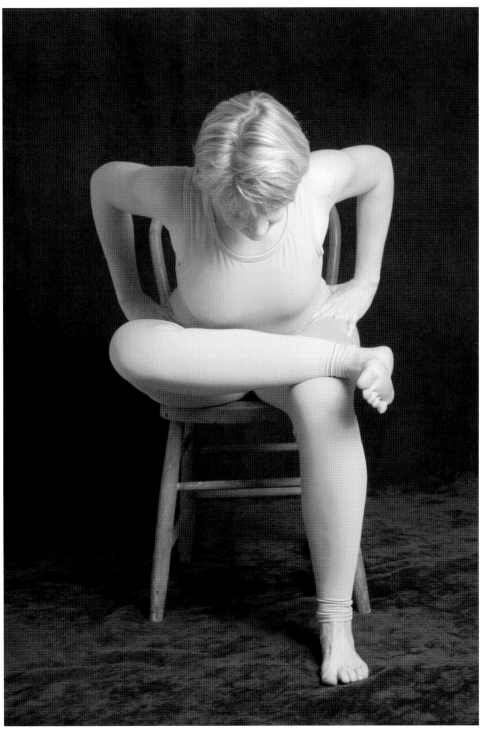

18 Seated Half Lotus preparation

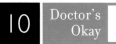

10 Doctor's Okay ☐

SEATED NECK STRETCH

After the effort of the first nine poses, this release for your neck muscles eases you back into stillness.

benefits
Stretches neck muscles

how to set up
Sit in Mountain. Soften your shoulders, your face, and your jaw. Rest your hands on your thighs. Rest in your steady *ujjayi* breath. Slowly drop your head to the right, aiming your right ear toward your shoulder. Enjoy a few breaths here.

on your inhalations and exhalations
Long, slow inhalations will slightly lift your neck and head out of the stretch a half inch or so. On your exhalations there will be more room to surrender into the stretch. Notice how your breath gently rocks your body, just as a loved one might gently cradle you in his or her arms.

to intensify
To deepen the stretch on the left side of your neck, lightly rest the fingertips of your right hand on the left side of your head. Hang your left arm down, as if you were carrying a heavy suitcase (photo 19).

to finish
Rest your hands in your lap and float your head back up through center. Then try the pose on the second side. Finally, sit quietly for a few minutes, simply breathing, simply being.

* * *

How do you feel after practicing the first sequence of yoga poses? Do you notice any subtle changes—physically, emotionally, and mentally? Does your breath feel easier?

Please observe your energy level. If you feel fatigued, I encourage you to enjoy five to twenty minutes in Resting Pose (p. 19). If you feel zippy, please continue on to the next chapter, *Ease*.

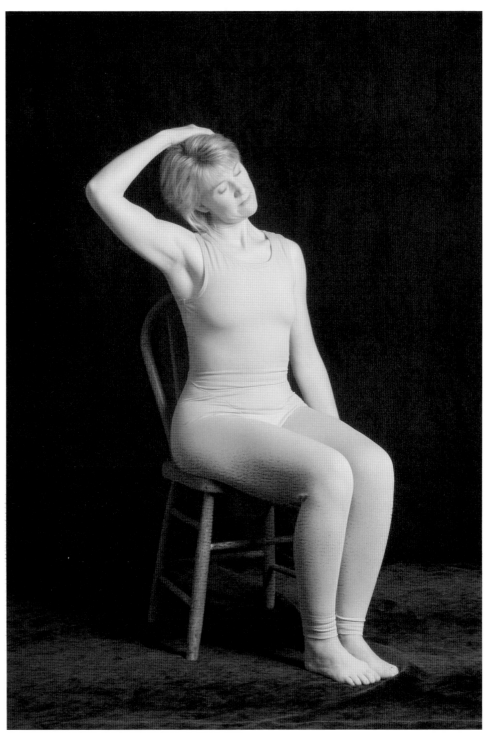

19 Seated Neck Stretch

CHAPTER 7

ease

While practicing yoga, you may wish to reflect on, "how is this like my life?" It can be powerful to observe how you approach your yoga practice. Are there subtle ways in which you treat yourself harshly? For instance, do you race through poses in order to complete the sequence quickly, or skip Resting Pose because it seems "unproductive," or berate yourself when you can't do the poses "perfectly"? Are you using yoga to try to conquer your body?

In my experience, one of the wonderful things about yoga is that your practice on the mat can be an experiment for your life off the mat. If you notice that you are not in the habit of being kind to yourself, if you hunger for ease and grace, try practicing yoga in ways that nourish and sus-

tain you. Take the time to explore and savor just a few poses, then be willing to stop and rest when you feel fatigued. Celebrate your every effort. In the space where you practice, surround yourself with beauty: a vase of fresh flowers, lit candles, photographs of loved ones, anything that makes you feel happy. Honor your body as the hardworking, resilient, sacred gift that it is.

In this sequence, you will work on a yoga mat.* So that you and your mat don't slip or slide, it is safest to place your yoga mat on an uncarpeted floor. If you wish to have extra padding underneath you, use neatly folded, firm blankets or towels on top of your mat. If you don't have a yoga mat this very minute, use a large towel on a carpeted floor instead.

---

*See *Resources* (p. 115) for information on ordering yoga equipment.

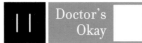

Doctor's Okay

RESTING CHILD
Vajrasana

When my son Benjamin was a tiny baby, he slept in Resting Child, completely relaxed and soft.

benefits
Releases lower back tension

how to set up
Come to hands and knees on your yoga mat or towel. Walk your knees back about twelve inches behind your hips. Place the tops of your feet on the ground with your toes long. Draw your hips back and down so that your buttocks rest close to your heels. If your belly or chest presses uncomfortably against your thighs, then widen your knees further apart to let your belly relax, and rest your forehead on your stacked fists (photo 20). Or, you may find greater ease in your neck if you extend your arms forward, palms and forehead resting on the ground (photo 21).

on your inhalations
Notice how your spacious, deep inhalations expand your back body.

on your exhalations
To invite greater ease into the pose, allow your body to have weight. Imagine being held up by the earth underneath you.

to finish
Shift forward onto hands and knees, and continue on to Yawning Dog.

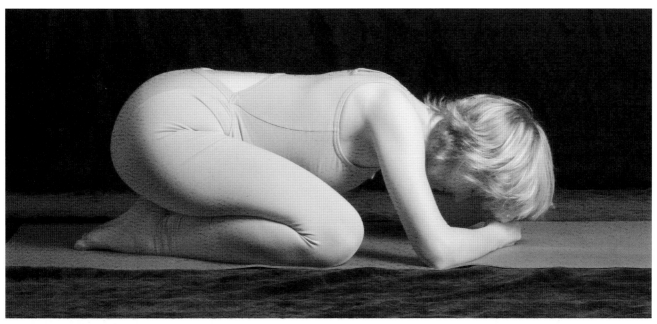

20 Resting Child variation I

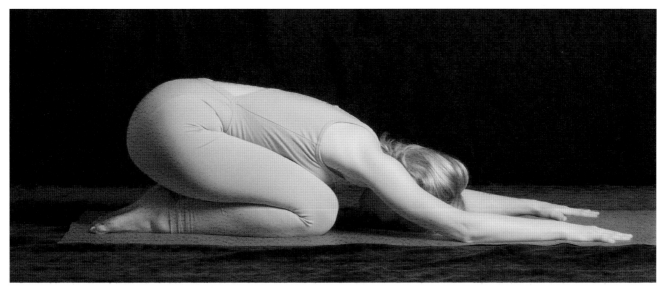

21 Resting Child variation II

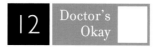
YAWNING DOG
Modified Adho Mukha Svanasana

Many yoga poses are inspired by animals, like Eagle, Crane, Peacock, Fish, Camel, Cobra, and Lion. This pose is a variation on Downward Facing Dog. Yawning optional!

benefits
Stretches sides of torso and back

how to set up
Come onto hands and knees. Place your palms on the ground directly underneath your shoulders, with fingers wide. Walk your knees back about twelve inches behind your hips. Curl your toes under, then draw your hips back and down so that your buttocks rest close to your heels. If your belly or chest presses uncomfortably against your thighs, widen your knees further apart.

To energize your arms, draw the head of your arm bones deeper into their shoulder joints. You will feel your shoulder blades press strongly onto your back. As you press your palms down, lift your forearms up toward the sky.

on your inhalations
When your breath is deep and slow, notice how your ribcage expands on your inhalations, so that your spine floats up toward the sky and your belly expands down against your thighs.

on your exhalations
Keep of the head of your arm bones deep into your shoulder joints and lengthen your spine. Reach your hips back as you creep your hands forward, like how a dog yawns and stretches (photo 22).

to intensify
Keep your hips anchored back and down, your arms energized, and now walk your torso and arms around to the right into a side bend. You will feel a marvelous stretch in your left armpit, ribcage, and waist (photo 23). To find ease here, as you curl to your right, breathe deeply so that the expansion and release of your lungs massage the muscles in your torso.

to finish
Creep your hands and torso back to center. Sit back on your heels and rest as needed. Notice if your left lung feels more spacious than your right lung! Try the pose on the second side, then continue on to Bow and Arrow.

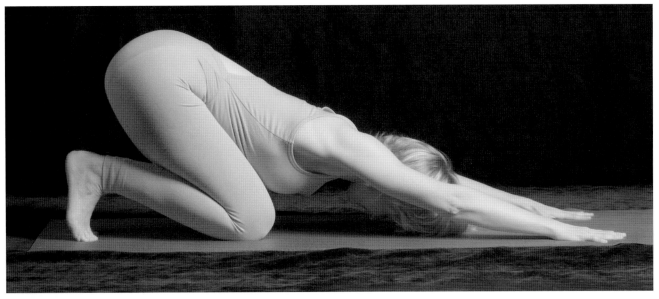

22 Yawning Dog variation I

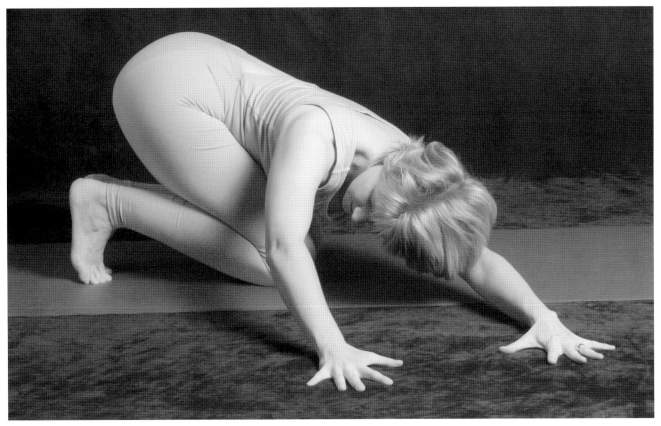

23 Yawning Dog variation II

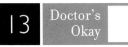

BOW AND ARROW
Modified Parighasana

To cultivate ease in yoga poses, I encourage you to give your best efforts, but not to force your body. In this satisfying twist, for instance, if you begin to feel strain in your neck or top shoulder, please use the suggested modifications as a way to honor your body.

benefits
Stretches chest, back and abdomen, squeezes and releases internal organs so that they are nourished with freshly oxygenated blood

how to set up
Once again shift forward onto hands and knees. Line up your shoulders directly over your hands and your hips directly over your knees. Come onto the tops of your fists so that your wrists are straight.

Draw the head of your arm bones deeply into your shoulder joints and firm your shoulder blades onto your back. As a result, your chest will drop a few inches closer toward the ground. Then, from the center of your chest and back, send energy down through your arms as if your knuckles could press deep into the earth. Firm your belly back toward your spine and expand your lower back wide and toward the sky, like bread dough rising.

After stabilizing your core body, extend your right leg out to the right, perpendicular to your torso, and place your right hand on your right hip. Begin a spinal twist: turn your torso to the right and up toward the sky. Gaze forward or down toward the ground to keep your neck relaxed (photo 24).

on your inhalations
You may notice that your body releases out of the spinal twist slightly on your inhalations.

on your exhalations
You may notice that there is suddenly room to twist more deeply on your exhalations. From the core of your body, spin your belly up toward the sky.

to intensify
Lead from the center of your chest to lift your right arm up toward the sky. Sweep your right arm back behind you, like an enormous wing (photo 25). If you feel any pinching in your right shoulder or chest, rest your right hand onto your waist again and turn more deeply from your torso.

to finish
Swoop your right arm back down and return to hands and knees. Pause in Resting Child (p. 44) as needed, then try the pose on the second side. Continue on to Pigeon.

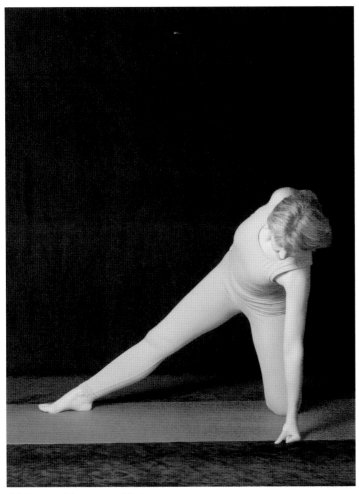

24 Bow and Arrow modified

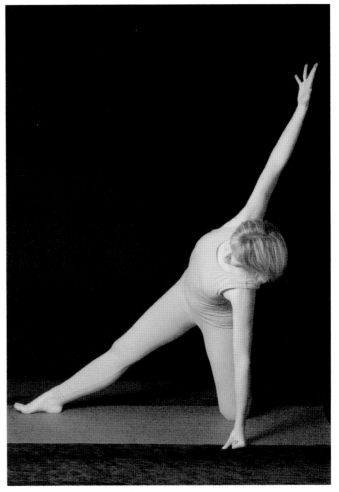

25 Bow and Arrow intensified

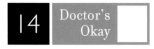

PIGEON

Modified Eka Pada Raja Kapotasana

The few times that I have injured myself in yoga class, it's been my ego that I've tripped over. Out of pride, I've tried to keep up with the teacher and didn't use discernment about what was appropriate for my body. So if you notice that you feel compelled to practice the "intensified" variation of each and every pose, then I encourage you pay attention to the truth of how your body feels in each pose, and from that truth, choose the variation that nurtures your body as it is today.

benefits

Stretches hips and legs

how to set up

Come onto hands and knees. Slide your right shin forward on the ground to bring your right knee next to your right thumb. Keep your right thigh directly over your right shin.

Tuck your left toes underneath so the balls of your left toes are on the ground. Keep your left knee on the ground. You will begin to feel a wonderful stretch in your right buttock and hip (photo 26).

on your inhalations

Notice if your pelvis has dropped down to the right. To find greater alignment here, float your pelvis up away from the ground a few inches, then draw the tops of your thighbones more deeply into their hip sockets. As you draw your right thigh *back*, and your left thigh *forward*, your hip bones will line up evenly across from one another.

on your exhalations

As you keep your pelvis stable, dive your tailbone straight down like an arrow toward the earth.

to intensify

If this is safe for your right knee, shift over to your right hip and slide your right shin forward, out from underneath your right thigh. Your right heel may rest in front of your left hip crease. Bring your pelvis back to center again. Now, fold forward from your hip creases as you keep your spine long and graceful. Rather than hunching your shoulders and bowing your head, slide your collarbones up toward the sky and wide like a bird spreading its wings to take flight. Rest your hands or forearms on the ground (photo 27).

to finish

Shift back onto hands and knees. Pause in Resting Child (p. 44) as needed, then try the pose on the second side. Continue on to Fire Log.

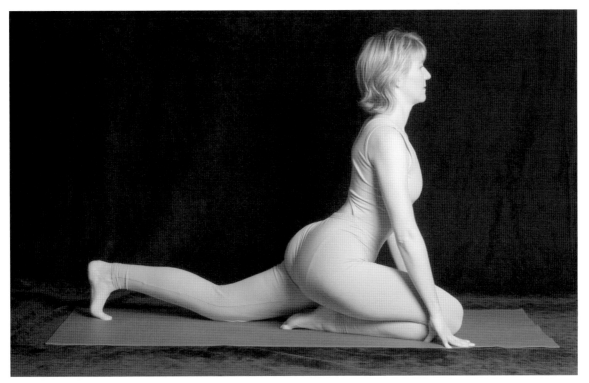

26 Pigeon modified

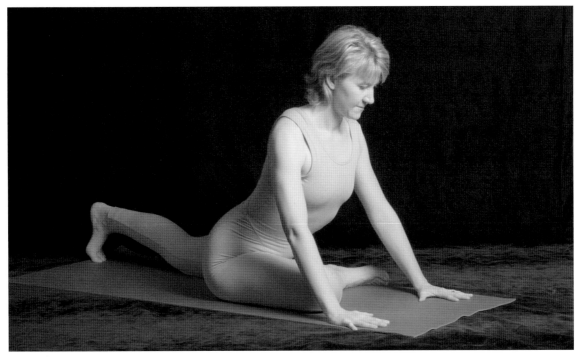

27 Pigeon intensified

FIRE LOG
Agnistambhasana

Fire Log is a wonderfully fiery stretch for your outer hips, so as you dive into the intensity of the pose, please also sustain a steady and deep ujjayi breath, relax your face, and rest your gaze on one spot on the ground. You know you're straining in a yoga pose when you find yourself frowning, gritting your teeth, or wildly looking around the room for the nearest exit!

benefits
Stretches hips, buttocks, and legs

how to set up
Sit cross-legged on your mat. Sit tall as in Seated Mountain (p. 22). Cross your right lower leg on top of your left lower leg like neatly stacking logs onto a woodpile. Place your right ankle directly on top of your left knee, so that your right foot hangs outside your left knee and you can wiggle your right foot freely. Slide your left lower leg forward on the ground so that your left ankle lines up directly underneath your right knee. Flex your feet strongly and widen your toes.

If you feel *any* pain in your knees, are tipped over onto one buttock, rounded in your spine, or are otherwise uncomfortable, please modify the pose. Cross your right ankle over your left ankle, press both sit bones into the ground (photo 28). If sitting on the ground is difficult, substitute Seated Half Lotus Preparation (p. 38) for this pose.

Now, with the head of your arm bones rolled back and your collarbones lifted and light, begin to fold forward from your hip creases (photo 29). These actions create a deep stretch in your buttocks and outer hips.

on your inhalations
You may notice that your torso rises up an inch or so out of the depth of the stretch.

on your exhalations
Fold more deeply. Allow yourself to melt into the heat and intensity of the stretch.

to finish
Slowly float your torso back upright, uncross your legs, extend your legs in front of you and wiggle them around a little to stretch out. Then try the pose on the second side. Continue on to Cobra.

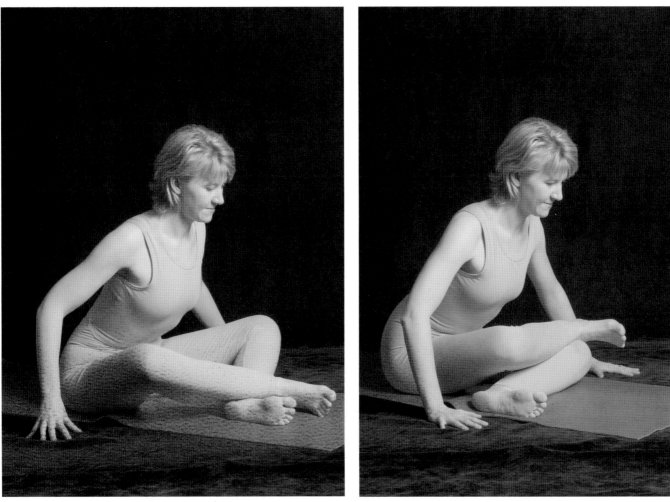

28 Fire Log modified

29 Fire Log intensified

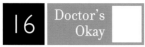

C O B R A
Bhujangasana

The next three backbends are fabulous: you will strengthen your back muscles, begin to reverse the effects of any habitual slumping or hunching over, and boost your energy and optimism. Here in Cobra, you might enjoy visualizing your spine in a long, graceful curve, easy and sinuous as a snake.

b e n e f i t s
Strengthens back, buttocks and legs, stretches chest

h o w   t o   s e t   u p
Lie on your belly with your hands next to the sides of your ribcage, palms on the ground, elbows bent and arms tucked in close to your torso. Bring your legs together. Widen your toes and press the tops of your feet and toes into the ground.

Roll your inner thighs up toward the sky: you will feel your buttocks lift slightly and the back of your pelvis widen as a result. Keep rolling your inner thighs up as you add the movement of sliding your tailbone back in the direction of your heels. In combination, these two movements will lengthen and stabilize your lower back: very important while practicing backbends. If you experience any pinching in your lower back during backbends, return and recommit to these actions.

Lightly shrug your shoulders up toward your ears, strongly back toward the back plane of your body, and press your shoulder blades magnetically onto your back. Now, float your head and chest up away from the ground (photo 30).

o n   y o u r   i n h a l a t i o n s
When your breath is spacious, notice how your torso bobs up a little on your inhale. Relax your face and jaw.

o n   y o u r   e x h a l a t i o n s
Use back strength to continue to arc up and back. Roll the head of your arm bones further back.

t o   i n t e n s i f y
Keep the stability in your lower back and now, without locking your elbows, use some arm strength to press up into a slightly deeper backbend. To strengthen your neck muscles without shortening the back of your neck, slide your skull back in space a few inches (photo 31).

t o   f i n i s h
Slowly lower your torso back down to the ground again. Turn your head to one side and rest your head on your hands. Let your whole body relax. Rest as needed, then continue on to Locust.

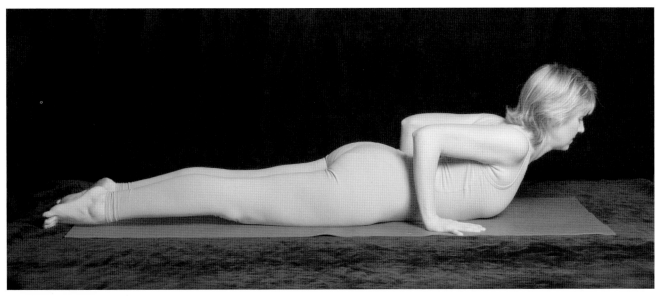

30 Cobra modified

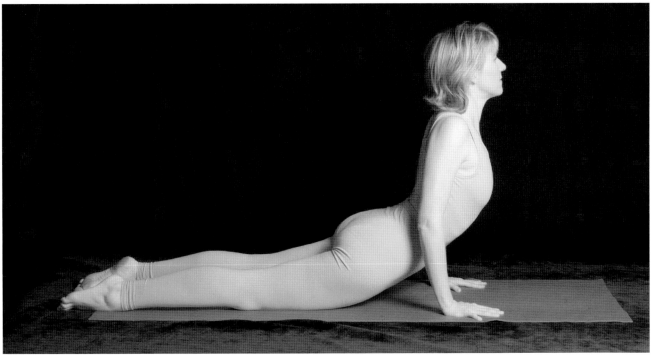

31 Cobra intensified

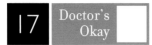

LOCUST
Salabhasana

Finding humor in challenging situations—and challenging yoga poses—helps me to cultivate a feeling of ease. In Locust, for example, I feel like a flying superhero from a comic book. Here come the yogis to save the day!

benefits
Strengthens back, buttocks and legs

how to set up
Come into Cobra again, then extend your arms back by your sides, parallel to the ground, palms facing one another. Roll the head of your arm bones strongly up and then back, away from the ground. With legs together and knees straight, lift your legs and torso up toward the sky (photo 32). As in Cobra, keep rolling your inner thighs up and lengthening your tailbone back so that your lower back does not compress.

on your inhalations
As in Cobra, with a full breath your torso will bob up and down.

on your exhalations
Lead from your inner thighs to lift the front of your legs further up away from the earth. Lead from the power of your upper back to lift higher into the backbend.

to intensify
If your back feels safe and strong, reach your arms out, like you're flying through the air! Up, up, and away! (photo 33)

to finish
Slowly release your arms and legs back down to the ground. Turn your head to one side and rest your head on your hands. Let your whole body relax. Rest as needed, then continue on to Bridge.

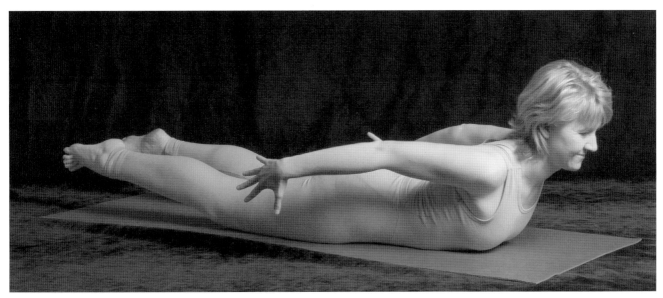

32 Locust modified

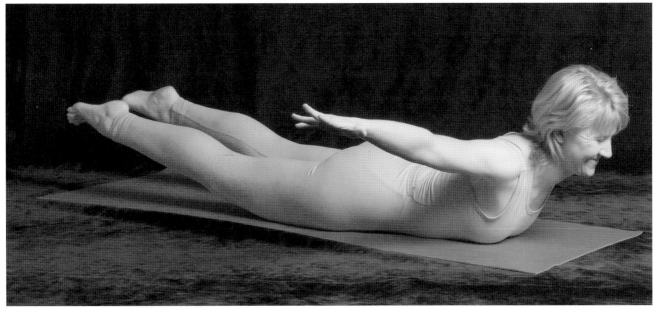

33 Locust intensified

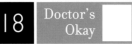
B R I D G E
Setu Bandhasana

To find ease in this powerful backbend, celebrate yourself on each breath. Commend yourself for your commitment, your stamina, and your willingness to try.

b e n e f i t s
Strengthens back and legs, stretches chest, abdomen, and front of thighs

h o w   t o   s e t   u p
Lie on your back with knees bent. Step your feet about six inches away from your buttocks. Place your feet flat on the ground, parallel to one another, and hips' width apart.

Take your arms down by your sides. Now bend your arms at right angles so that the back of your upper arms press into the earth and your fingers point toward the sky. Lightly shrug your shoulders up in the direction of your head, then strongly roll the head of your arm bones back, and root them to the ground. You will feel the muscles around your shoulder blades strengthen, like friendly hands supporting the lift of your heart.

o n   y o u r   i n h a l a t i o n s
Imagine your breath creating more space in your chest for your big, generous heart to expand into.

o n   y o u r   e x h a l a t i o n s
Strongly press down with your upper arms. From the strength of your upper back, lift your chest up toward the sky. Arch your upper back away from the ground, enough so that a toy race car could zoom through the space between your upper back and the ground (photo 34).

t o   i n t e n s i f y
Lift your chest victoriously and float your hips up. Press down strongly with your lower legs and feet into the earth. Extend your arms down by your sides, heads of your arm bones rolled back and down toward the earth, palms facing up. Lengthen your tailbone in the direction of your knees.

When your torso and pelvis feel buoyant, tuck one shoulder at a time under your torso, like tucking in sheets under a mattress. Clasp your hands together (photo 35) or hold a strap between your hands.

t o   f i n i s h
Release your arms and slowly roll down your spine. Hug your knees to your chest and rest as needed, then continue on to Fountain.

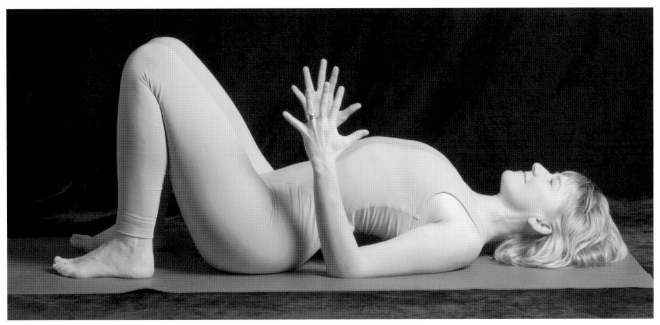

34 Bridge modified

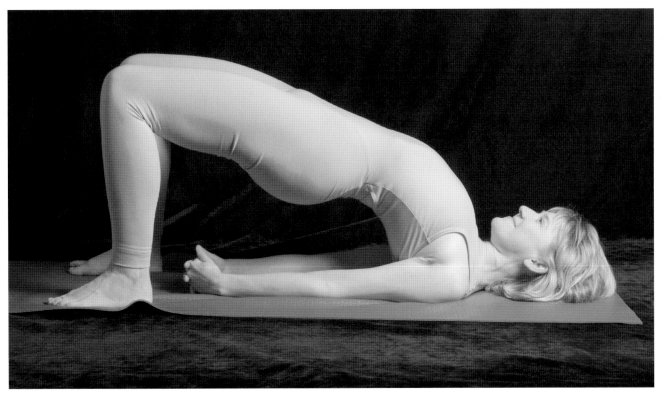

35 Bridge intensified

FOUNTAIN
Supta Hasta Padangusthasana

Using your imagination is yet another way to find both ease and depth in yoga poses. I notice that people's bodies respond not just to technical explanations but also to poetic suggestions. In Fountain, I suggest watery images, but you may prefer, for instance, to visualize your legs like shiny blades of a Swiss Army knife, straight and sturdy.

benefits
Stretches lower back and legs

how to set up
Lie on your back with knees bent. Step your feet a comfortable distance away from your buttocks. Place your feet flat on the ground, parallel to one another, and hips' width apart.

To arch your lower back off the ground, rock the front of your pelvis forward, in the direction of your feet. Extend your left leg long on the ground. When your lower back is in an exaggerated arch, then the back of your left leg will press strongly into the ground, creating a steady foundation for the rest of the pose.

Now bring your lower back into its natural curve again: keep the back of your left leg grounded. Slide the sides of your ribcage down toward the earth. Lengthen your tailbone in the direction of your left foot.

As the back of your left leg, your hips, and your torso are firmly grounded, bring your right knee into your chest. Clasp your hands around the back of your right thigh and extend your right leg up toward the sky. If your shoulders hunch up off the floor, use a strap or long towel behind your thigh instead (photo 36).

on your inhalations
Stabilize your body: roll the head of your arm bones back toward the ground, which will widen and lift your chest. Roll your left inner thigh down toward the earth so that your left toes and knee face the sky. Flex your feet and widen your toes. As you stabilize, envision yourself as solid as the earth itself.

on your exhalations
Energize your body: extend out through your left leg like a rushing stream as you reach your right leg up to the sky and toward your head, like a fountain shooting up and spilling over (photo 37).

to finish
Release your hands, hug both knees to your chest, and try the pose on the second side. Continue on to Bug to rest.

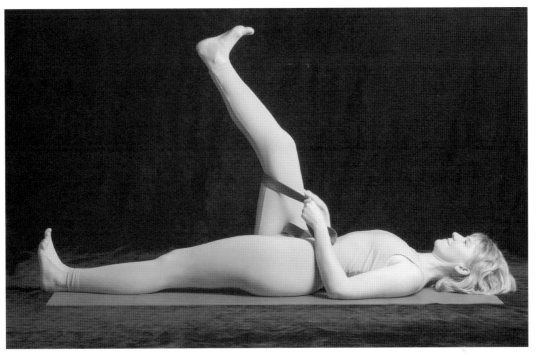

36 Fountain modified

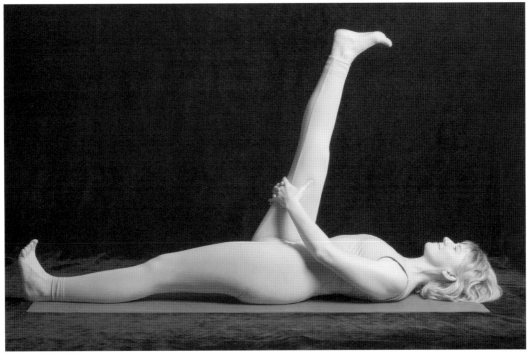

37 Fountain intensified

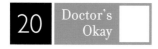

BUG

Remember the phrase "snug as a bug in a rug"? As you rest comfortably in Bug, please enjoy the effects of the yoga poses that you have practiced.

benefits
Gently stretches back muscles

how to set up
Lie on your back and hug your knees to your chest. Clasp your hands behind your thighs or around the front of your shins to help you snuggle your legs closer to your torso. If your shoulders hunch up off the floor, hold a yoga strap or towel behind your thighs instead, so that the back of your shoulders can rest on the ground (photo 38).

on your inhalations
Notice how your inhales create expansion in your core body: your lower back presses down into the ground, your belly presses out against your thighs, and the sides of your ribcage widen.

on your exhalations
Keep your face and jaw relaxed as you bring your thighs closer to your chest (photo 39).

to intensify
Deepen your *ujjayi* breath. The expansion and release of your breath will gently massage your lower back.

to finish
Release your arms and step your feet to the ground.

***

If you feel energized, please continue on to the next chapter, *Strength*. Or, if you feel fatigued, I invite you to stretch out in Resting Pose (p. 19) for five to twenty minutes.

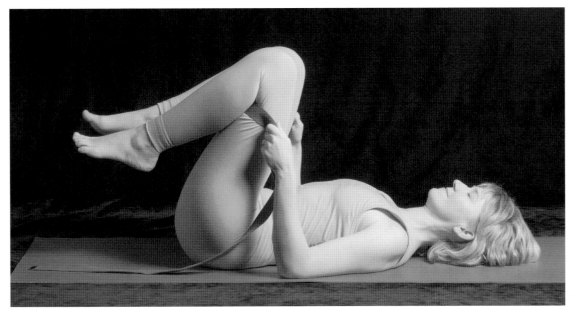

38 Bug modified

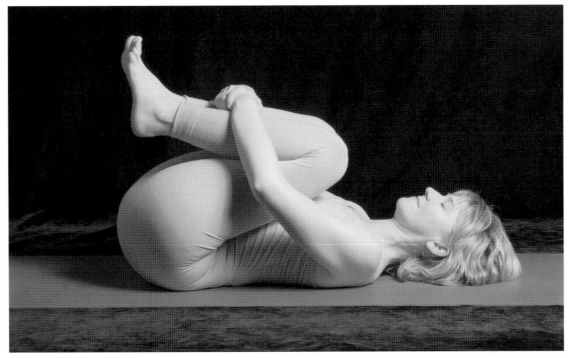

39 Bug intensified

strength

When life gets hard, what are your sources of inner strength? Perhaps the love of your family and friends? Perhaps your faith? Sheer determination? I invite you to visualize or meditate on your sources of strength as you practice this ambitious sequence. In doing so, you create physical memories of yourself as resilient, infuse your efforts with personal meaning, and resonate with sources of strength greater than just your own individual efforts—the power of love, the gift of grace, the dignity of being part of the grand sweep of humanity.

As you work on strengthening your core body, please incorporate the self-honoring practices that you cultivated throughout the sequence *Ease*. I encourage you to use discernment: if a pose is too strenuous for your body today, please skip it or choose the modified variation. Seek a balance between ease and effort, so that you leave your yoga practice refreshed rather than exhausted.

In this sequence, you will work on your yoga mat. So that you and your mat don't slip or slide, it is safest to place your yoga mat on an uncarpeted floor. If you would like padding to lie upon for poses 21–25, or underneath your knees for poses 26–30, use neatly folded, firm blankets or towels on top of your mat. If you don't have a yoga mat, use a large towel on a carpeted floor instead.

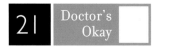
PELVIC TILT

Slowly rocking back and forth in Pelvic Tilt is not only a warm-up for the abdominal and back strengthening work in this sequence, but also a marvelous massage for your lower back.

benefits
Releases lower back tension, tones abdomen

how to set up
Lie on your back with knees bent. Step your feet a comfortable distance away from your buttocks. Place your feet flat on the ground, parallel to one another, and hips' width apart.

Extend your arms out wide, at shoulder height, with palms facing up and fingers spread wide. As in Seated Wings (p. 28), lightly shrug your shoulders up in the direction of your head, then strongly roll the head of your arm bones back and root them to the ground. You will feel the muscles around your shoulder blades strengthen so that your shoulder blades snuggle onto your back.

Remember to keep your foundation strong: toes wide and lifted, feet grounded, and arms rooted into the earth.

on your inhalations
Rock the front of your pelvis forward, in the direction of your feet. Notice that your lower back *arches away* from the earth as a result. Arch enough so that a toy race car could zip through the space between your lower back and the ground (photo 40).

on your exhalations
Rock the front of your pelvis back, in the direction of your head. Notice that your lower back lengthens and *expands into* the earth as a result. Expand enough so that the toy race car could not fit between your back and the ground (photo 41). Lengthen your buttocks toward your knees rather than clenching your buttock muscles.

to intensify
Use your core body strength to slow the movements down: imagine rolling along your spine one vertebra at a time. Stay in each shape—arching, expanding—for a few long breaths. Luxuriate in the lovely release in your back and neck muscles.

to finish
Rest in Bug (p. 62) as needed, then continue on to Bowl.

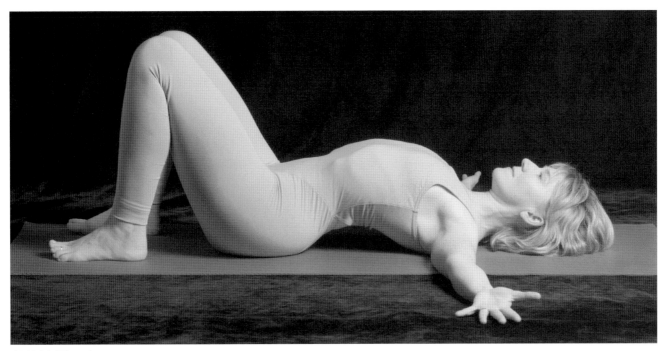

40 Pelvic Tilt arch

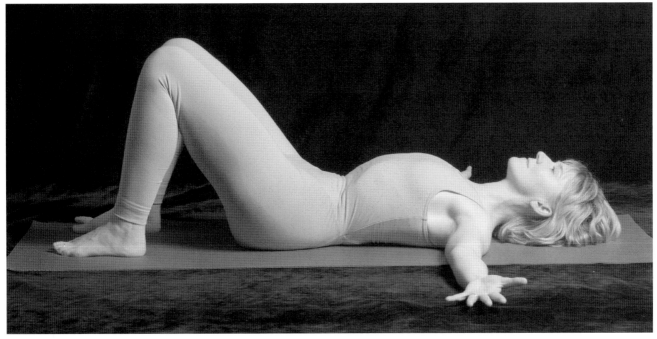

41 Pelvic Tilt expansion

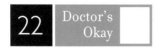

BOWL

Going through hard times sometimes requires me to be stronger and more adaptable than I think myself capable of. Similarly, as the variations on Bowl become increasingly challenging, you may discover that you have more grit and strength than you imagine.

benefits
Strengthens abdomen, releases back tension

how to set up
Lie on your back with knees bent. Step your feet a comfortable distance away from your buttocks. Place your feet flat on the ground, parallel to one another, and hips' width apart.

Interlace your fingers behind your head and rest your head in your hands on the ground. Now, without using the strength of your leg or buttock muscles, draw your pubic bone and the front of your ribcage toward one another. Notice that your lower back presses into the earth as a result, just like the expanding movement in Pelvic Tilt (p. 66).

on your inhalations
Relax the muscles in your face and jaw.

on your exhalations
Without clenching your buttock muscles or pressing your feet down into the earth, roll your tailbone further up toward the sky to shorten the distance between the front of your pelvis and your ribcage.

to intensify
1. Float the soles of your feet a half-inch off the ground, as if you didn't want to leave any footprints. It is normal for your abdominal muscles to shake.
2. Roll your head and upper back up off the ground. So that you don't strain your neck, keep your elbows wide and allow your head to be heavy like a bowling ball in your hands (photo 42). Roll more of your spine up off the ground rather than pulling on your head with your hands.
3. Place a yoga block or rolled up towel between your inner thighs. Extend your legs toward the sky with flexed feet. If you need to keep your knees bent, that's fine. Squeeze into the block with your inner thighs. Roll your tailbone up toward the sky. For greater intensity, slowly take your legs a few inches further away from your head.
4. Combine variations 2 and 3: Now roll both ends of your spine up off the ground, similar to the shape of a shallow bowl (photo 43).

to finish
Rest in Bug (p. 62) as needed, then continue on to Twist.

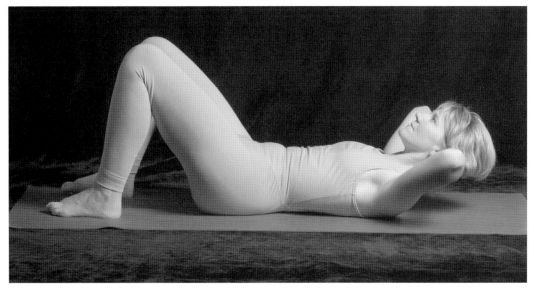

42 Bowl modified

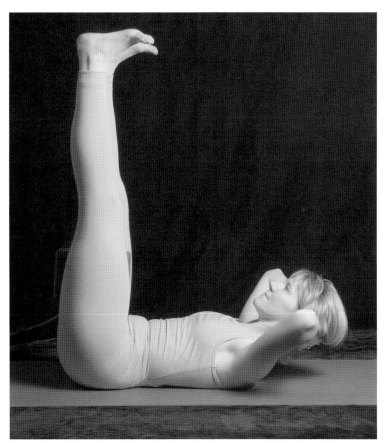

43 Bowl intensified

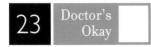

TWIST

Modified Jathara Parivartanasana

For me, a gift of going through hard times has been discovering how much support is available to me. For instance, at a time when I was grieving a death, I also was deeply moved by my community's generosity and tenderness toward me. Both experiences were true at once.

This twist embodies turning toward your faith or your loved ones, present or past. As you come out of the twist, back to your center, imagine bringing their gifts of love with you, into the truth of the present moment.

benefits

Stretches back and outer hips, squeezes and releases internal organs so that they are nourished with freshly oxygenated blood

how to set up

Lie on your back and hug your knees to your chest. Extend your arms out wide, at shoulder height, with palms facing up and fingers spread wide. Lightly shrug your shoulders up in the direction of your head, then strongly roll the head of your arm bones back, and root them to the ground. Like great wings spreading wide, press down into the earth through your upper back and arms all the way out to your fingers.

Keep your whole wingspan grounded and now slowly lower your knees to the right, about halfway to the ground. Aim your knees in the direction of your right elbow. Flex your feet strongly. Turn your torso and gaze to the left, into a spinal twist, toward your sources of strength (photo 44).

on your inhalations

Invite your breath to be spacious and full. You may notice that you come out of the depth of the twist an inch or two on your inhalations.

on your exhalations

Turn your torso more deeply to the left. Only go as far as you can keep both shoulder blades firmly rooted on the ground.

to intensify

Float your legs even closer to the earth, so that the outside of your right leg and foot just barely graze the ground. Or straighten your left leg so your left foot extends toward your right hand (photo 45).

to finish

On an inhalation, slowly float your legs back up through center.

Step your feet to the ground. Rest for a few breaths, allowing the effects of the deep twist to soak in. Then try the pose on the second side. Try both sides a few times, then continue on to Scissors.

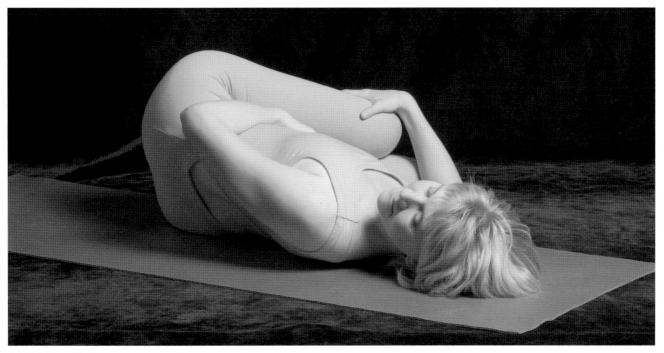

44 Twist modified

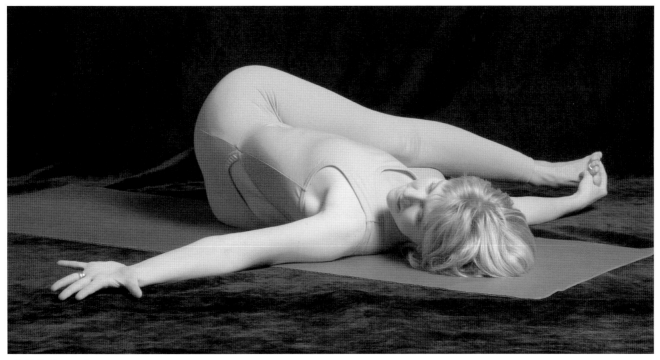

45 Twist intensified

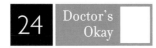

SCISSORS
Modified Urdhva Prasarita Padasana

Sometimes, what takes the greatest strength is to stay centered and quiet, to be at the eye of the storm. Similarly, in this pose it takes determination to stay grounded as you slowly lower and lift one or both legs.

benefits
Strengthens abdomen, back, and legs

how to set up
Lie on your back with your knees bent. Step your feet a comfortable distance away from your buttocks. Place your feet flat on the ground.

Interlace your hands behind your head and rest your head in your hands on the ground. As in Bowl (p. 68), draw the front of your pelvis and the front of your ribcage toward one another so your belly feels strong. Expand and widen your lower back into the earth.

Extend your right leg up toward the sky. Flex your right foot and widen your toes. Now slowly lower your right leg down as far as you can maintain stability in your belly and lower back (photo 46). Rather than clenching your buttock muscles, lengthen your tailbone up toward the sky. Lighten the sole of your left foot as if you don't want to leave a footprint.

on your inhalations
Seek ease, even as you work hard. Relax your face and jaw. Take refuge in your *ujjayi* breath.

on your exhalations
Stay still in your core body, so that your lower back doesn't overarch and your legs don't suddenly plop down. After a few long breaths, slowly float your right leg back up to the sky. Hug both knees to your chest to rest, then try the pose on the second side.

to intensify
Extend both legs up toward the sky, legs together, feet flexed, and toes wide. Keep the quiet stability in your core body as you slowly begin to lower both legs (photo 47). After a few long breaths, slowly float your legs back up toward the sky.

to finish
Hug your knees to your chest. Rest in Bug (p. 62) as needed, then continue on to Bow.

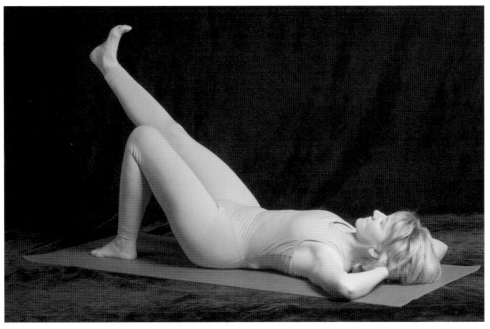

46 Scissors modified

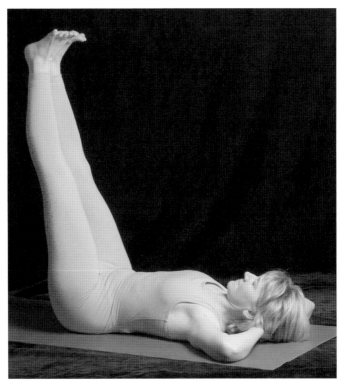

47 Scissors intensified

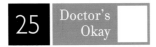
B O W
Dhanurasana

The stronger you are in this backbend, the higher your heart will rise, and the more exposed your chest may feel. Envision your sources of inner strength collectively lifting you up, supporting you in being fully alive in this moment, open and vulnerable to all of its joy and beauty and heartbreak.

benefits
Strengthens back, buttocks and legs, stretches chest and abdomen

how to set up
Lie on your belly. Rest your head on your left forearm. Bend your right knee and catch your right ankle with your right hand. Flex your right foot strongly. If these actions create *any* pain in your right knee, please use a yoga strap (or long towel) around your ankle rather than your hand (photo 48).

Lengthen and stabilize your lower back: roll your inner thighs up and lengthen your tailbone back, as in Cobra (p. 54). Bring your right heel in the direction of your right buttock. These actions create a deep stretch in the front of your right thigh.

After several long breaths, release your right ankle and slowly bring your leg to the ground. Try the pose on the second side.

to intensify
Now bend both knees and grasp both ankles with your hands or with your strap or towel. Flex both feet and widen your toes. Stabilize your lower back first, then draw your lower legs back, in the direction of the wall behind you. Press the front of your thighs deep into the ground. As a result, the front of your torso will begin to rise up off the ground (photo 49). Keep your knees in line with your hips rather than allowing your knees to splay wide.

on your inhalations
In response to your *ujjayi* breathing, your body may rock forward and back in this pose.

on your exhalations
Draw your lower legs further back to rise up high and triumphant in your heart.

to finish
Slowly release your ankles and float your arms, legs and torso back down to the ground. Turn your head to one side and rest your head on your hands. Let your whole body relax. Rest as needed, then continue on to Sleep Walker.

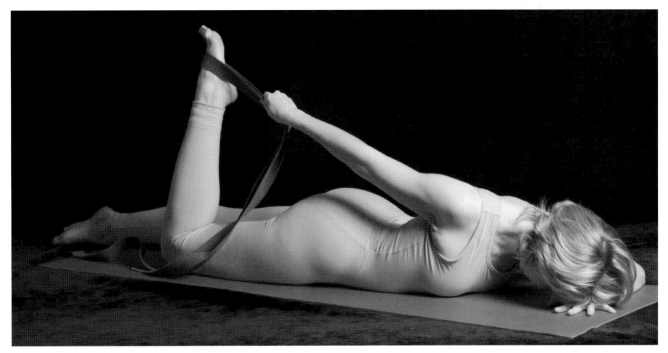

48 Bow modified

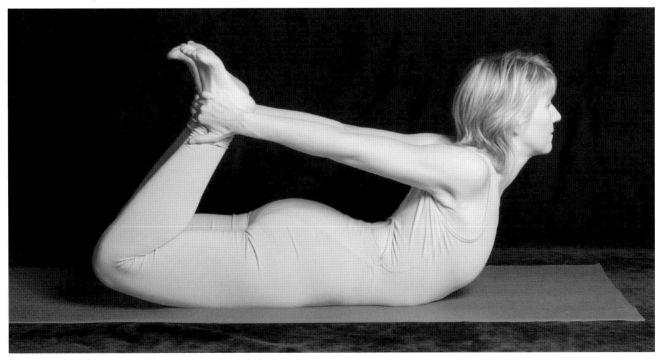

49 Bow intensified

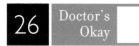

S L E E P W A L K E R

In Sleepwalker, you prepare for the final three strengthening poses. Extend your arms out from your radiant heart and reach beyond any barriers to living passionately and truthfully.

b e n e f i t s
Strengthens upper back, tones abdomen

h o w   t o   s e t   u p
Sit comfortably—cross-legged, on your heels, or in a chair. Extend your arms in front of you, palms facing forward and fingers spread wide.

Lightly shrug your shoulders up, strongly roll the head of your arm bones back, and draw your shoulder blades magnetically onto your back. As a result, the head of your arms will draw back into their shoulder joints and your chest will naturally lift.

o n   y o u r   i n h a l a t i o n s
Relax your face. Notice how your breath expands your chest, floating your collarbones up and wide.

Snuggle the head of your arm bones even deeper into their shoulder joints.

o n   y o u r   e x h a l a t i o n s
Keep the head of your arm bones deep into their shoulder joints, and on your exhales extend out from your chest and back, through your arms, as if pushing open a huge door in front of you (photo 50).

So that you don't overarch your lower back, slide the sides of your ribcage back toward the wall behind you and lengthen your tailbone down toward the earth. As a result, your lower back will feel expansive and full, as in Pelvic Tilt (p. 66).

Like a gentle hug, firm your belly back toward your spine. As a result, the front of your ribcage and pubic bone will reach toward one another, as in Bowl (p. 68).

t o   f i n i s h
Release your arms and rest with your hands on your thighs. Continue on to Balance Beam.

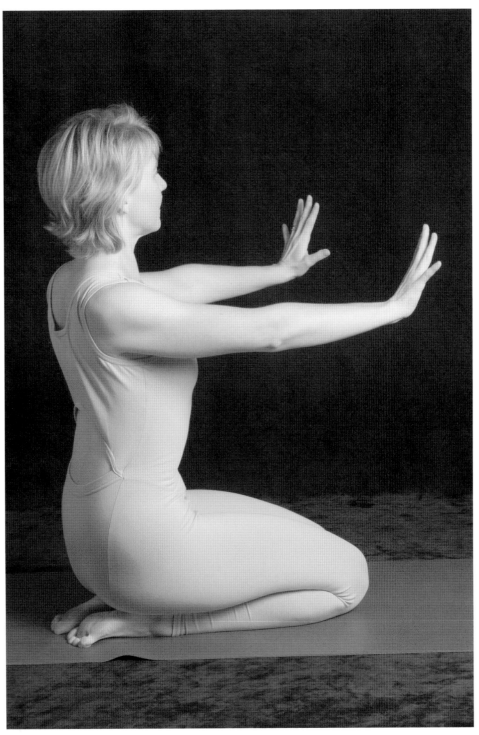

50 Sleepwalker

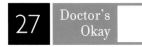

BALANCE BEAM

It takes inner strength to kindly say no to opinions, commitments, or relationships that deplete you, and instead to steadily focus your precious time and energy on what nourishes you. Similarly, this pose appears simple, but requires a firm intention to stabilize your core body.

benefits
Strengthens abdomen, back, buttocks and legs

how to set up
Shift forward onto all fours with your hands lined up directly underneath your shoulders and your knees lined up directly underneath your hips. If your wrists feel tender, instead of placing your palms onto the ground, rest the tops of your fists on the ground so that your wrists are straight.

As in Sleep Walker (p. 76), draw the head of your arm bones deeply into your shoulder joints and firm your shoulder blades onto your back. As a result, your chest will drop a few inches closer to the ground. Then, from your heart, extend energy out all the way through your hands and deep into the earth. As a result, your arms will strengthen and lengthen. Firm your belly back toward your spine and expand your lower back wide and up toward the sky.

Keep your core body still, and now slowly extend your right arm forward and up, thumb side of your hand facing up. Extend your left leg back with your foot strongly flexed and balls of your toes on the ground. Keep your head in line with your spine (photo 51).

on your inhalations
Stabilize: draw the head of your right arm bone more deeply into its joint as you roll your biceps up toward the sky and triceps down toward the earth. Roll your left inner thigh up toward the sky so that your left knee and toes roll down to face the earth.

on your exhalations
Energize: from your heart, extend your right arm further and lift it higher. Reach out boldly, and at the same time, don't collapse in your core body.

to intensify
Now float your left foot off the ground so that, without lifting your left hip, your left leg begins to come parallel to the earth. Seek stillness at your core. Slide the sides of your ribcage up toward the sky so that your lower back feels expansive and your abdomen feels strong (photo 52).

to finish
Slowly float your right arm and left leg down, back to all fours. Now try the pose on the second side: left arm and right leg lift up. Pause in Resting Child (p. 44) as needed, then continue on to Plank.

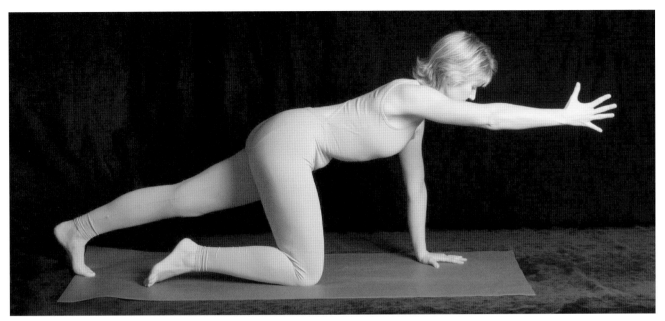

51 Balance Beam modified

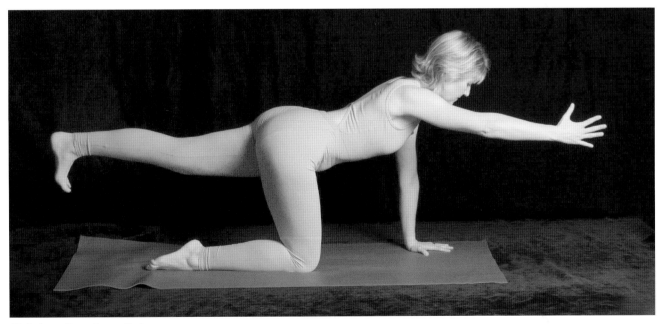

52 Balance Beam intensified

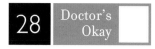

PLANK
Modified Chatturanga Dandasana

When holding Plank gets hard, when you want to give up, I invite you to focus on each spacious, smooth breath, one at a time. Bring to mind your sources of inner strength, as if you are being lightly held up in this pose by the powers of love and grace and mercy.

benefits
Builds arm, chest, back, and abdominal strength

how to set up
From hands and knees, come down onto your forearms with your elbows shoulder width apart and palms facing down, fingers wide. Bring your shoulders directly over your elbows and your hips over your knees.

Draw the head of your arm bones deeply into your shoulder sockets and firm your shoulder blades onto your back. As a result, your chest will drop a few inches closer toward the ground. Then, from your heart, extend energy out through your arms, as if you could sink your forearms and palms deep into the earth, like warm knives through butter. As a result, your arms will strengthen and lengthen. Firm your belly back toward your spine and expand your lower back wide and up toward the sky.

Without lifting your hips up, step your right leg long behind you, balls of your toes on the ground. Strengthen your right leg: stretch your heel back toward the wall behind you and lift your inner thigh up toward the sky. Then, without moving your pelvis at all, step your left leg back. If this is too strenuous, bring your knees to the ground (photo 53).

on your inhalations
If your breath suddenly becomes small and shallow, deepen and lengthen your inhalations.

on your exhalations
Stay solid and quiet at your core: Slide the sides of your ribcage up toward the sky and your tailbone back toward your heels so that your lower back feels expansive and your abdomen feels strong (photo 54).

to finish
Come back onto all fours. Pause in Resting Child (p. 44) as needed, then continue on to Gate.

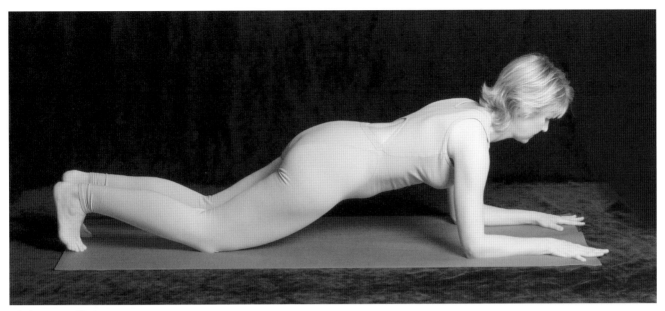

53 Plank modified

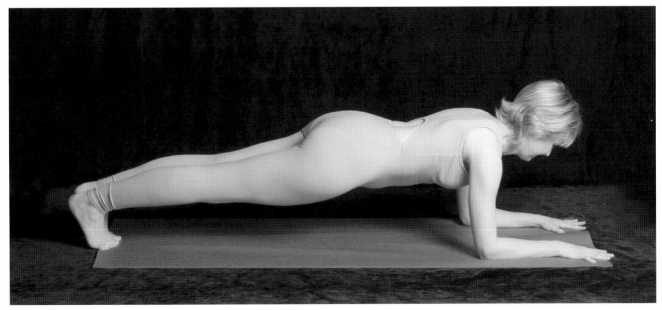

54 Plank intensified

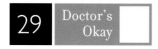

GATE
Parighasana

Gate is an advanced variation of Bow and Arrow (p. 48). It takes strength to find the lightness and playfulness in this challenging pose. Just like life!

benefits
Strengthens back and abdomen, lengthens sides of waist, stretches chest, squeezes and releases internal organs so that they are nourished with freshly oxygenated blood

how to set up
Start by standing on your knees. Take your right leg out to the right, in line with your right hip. If it is uncomfortable to bring the sole of your right foot onto the ground, then keep your heel on the ground and rest the balls of your right foot on the wall or a yoga block.

Take your hands to your hip creases. Shift your hips to the left and lengthen your torso to the right, directly over your right leg. Begin a spinal twist: root your tailbone and turn your torso up toward the sky. Keep your gaze down toward the ground (photo 55).

on your inhalations
You may notice that your body releases out of the spinal twist slightly on your inhalations.

on your exhalations
You may notice that there is suddenly room to twist more deeply on your exhalations. From the core of your body, spin your belly up toward the sky.

to intensify
Without shifting your hips back behind you, slide your right hand down your right shin. Sweep your left arm overhead and in the direction of your right foot. Now float your right arm up, off your leg, toward your left arm (photo 56). Lightly hover in space.

to finish
On an inhalation, float your torso back up through center and your arms down by your side. Try the pose on the second side, then continue on to Repose to rest.

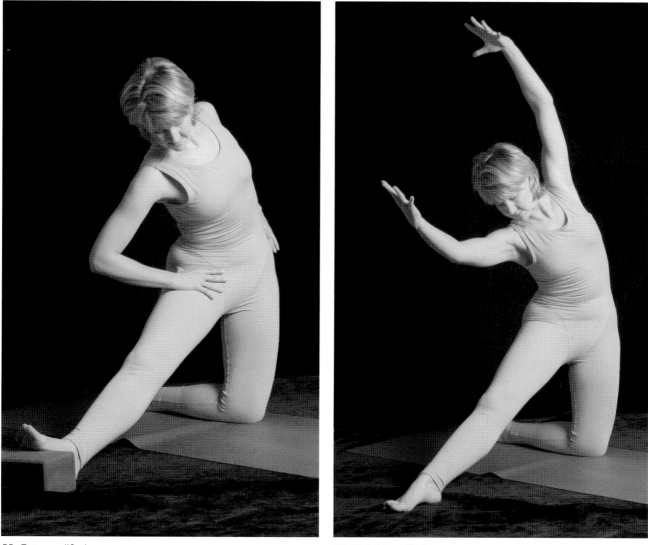

55 Gate modified

56 Gate intensified

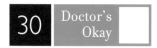
REPOSE
Modified Virasana

After working so powerfully, please savor the tranquility of resting in Repose.

benefits
Creates a comfortable place to rest

how to set up
From all fours, sit back on your heels with the top of your feet on the ground and toes long. If your knees complain, use props to sit higher. Place a folded blanket or yoga mat between the back of your thighs and your calves (photo 57). If you still feel any discomfort, please pause in Resting Child (p. 44) or stretch out in Resting Pose (p. 19) instead.

Rest your hands easily on your thighs with your elbows slightly bent. Sit with dignity (photo 58).

on your inhalations
Enjoy the gentle expansion of your spacious lungs.

Breathe into the full circumference of your ribcage: inhale into your back ribs, your front ribs, and into the sides of your ribcage.

on your exhalations
Invite your whole body to relax. You might imagine your shoulder blades, arm bones, and collarbones like a heavy velvet cloak resting on the regal and strong core of your body.

* * *

Again, please observe your energy level. If, after a few minutes of rest in Repose, you feel energized, continue on to the final chapter, *Courage*. If you are weary, I encourage you to make yourself completely comfortable in Resting Pose for five to twenty minutes.

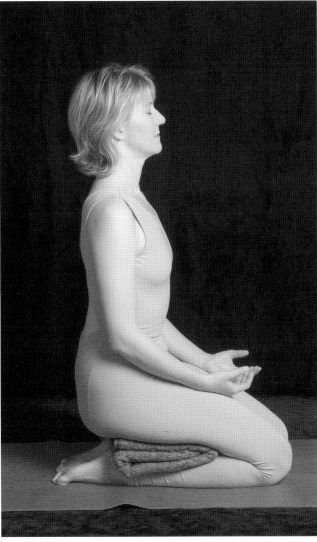

57 Repose modified

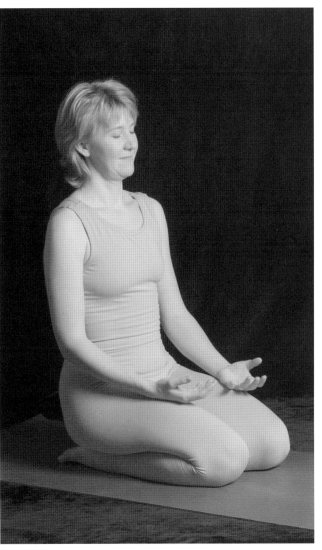

58 Repose intensified

courage

Standing poses embody determination and confidence: you literally stand on your own two feet. Engaging the muscles in your feet and legs establishes a foundation from which your spine lengthens, your heart lifts, and your arms extend.

What will you take a stand for? What is at the hot core of your fierce passion for life? In this final sequence of poses, I invite you to courageously take a stand for all that brings you love, sparks your enthusiasm, and sustains your passion.

In this sequence, you will work on your mat near a wall. So that you and your mat don't slip or slide, it is safest to place your yoga mat on an uncarpeted floor. If you don't have a yoga mat, work barefoot on an uncarpeted floor.

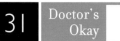

MOUNTAIN
Tadasana

As you integrate the principles of Mountain, you will move with greater ease, length, and grace. Try this pose as you're taking a walk or waiting in line.

benefits
Supports muscular and skeletal alignment

how to set up
Stand with your feet hips' width apart and parallel to one another. As in Seated Mountain (p. 22), lift and spread your toes, press down and wide through the four "corners" of your feet: the mound of your big toe, inner heel, outer heel, and mound of your little toe. Working your feet in this manner will strengthen every one of your yoga poses.

Place a yoga block or firmly rolled up towel between your inner thighs. Press down especially through your inner heels as you sweep your inner thighs back and wide. As a result, the block or towel will move back in space, and you may feel like you're sticking out your bottom. The action of bringing your thighbones back and wide expands the back of your pelvis (photo 59).

Keep the back of your pelvis broad, and now slide your tailbone down toward the earth (photo 60). As a result, you will feel your inner thighs grip the block, your lower back lengthen, your pubic bone tip up, your abdomen firm toward your spine, and your feet and legs connect more solidly to the earth. (And your bottom isn't sticking out anymore.)

If the block juts forward when you anchor your tailbone down, you are probably clenching your buttock muscles or curling your tailbone under. Rather than squeezing your buttocks together, lengthen straight down, as if you had a very heavy dinosaur tail dropping down to the ground.

Here's a subtle distinction to strengthen your legs and avoid hyperextension in your knee joints: as your thighs continue to move back, resist your shins and calves forward.

on your inhalations
With your toes still lifted and spread, imagine inhaling energy up from the molten core of the earth, through your feet, and up into your pelvis as you sweep your inner thighs back and wide.

on your exhalations
Extend downward: imagine exhaling energy from your pelvis back down through your tailbone, down through your legs, down through the four corners of your feet, down through all ten toes, and deep into the ground.

to finish
When you feel solid in Mountain, please continue to Mountain Top.

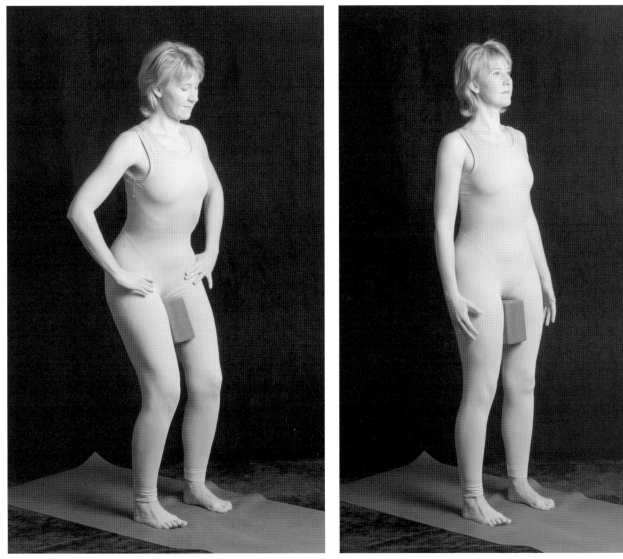

59 Mountain preparation

60 Mountain with block

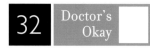

MOUNTAIN TOP
Urdhva Hastasana

In Mountain Top, you both root deeply into the earth and extend upward toward the sky, like you're ten miles tall.

benefits
Supports muscular and skeletal alignment

how to set up
Now, without using the yoga block, please stand tall in Mountain. Are your feet still lively? Can you still find the subtle balance of sweeping your inner thighs back and wide *and* lengthening your tailbone down?

Lightly shrug your shoulders up, strongly roll the head of your arm bones back, and draw your shoulder blades firmly onto your back. You will feel aliveness and strength in your upper back and a lift in your heart. Extend your arms straight in front of you. Draw the head of your arm bones deeper into their shoulder joints (photo 61) as in Sleepwalker (p. 76). Then sweep your arms overhead, as far as your range of motion allows today, with your palms facing one another (photo 62).

Also as in Sleepwalker, add core body strength: slide the sides of your ribcage an inch or two back in space so that your belly tones and your lower back widens. Even as you are working strongly, soften your face and jaw, and smooth out your breath.

on your inhalations
Recommit to drawing the head of your arm bones deep into their shoulder joints. When you do, you will create more space between your shoulders and ears. Instead of clenching up, the top of your shoulders will stay relaxed.

on your exhalations
Energize and lengthen out through your arms and hands, as if stars could shoot from your fingertips.

to finish
Slowly release your arms down by your sides. Rest as needed, then continue on to Right Angle.

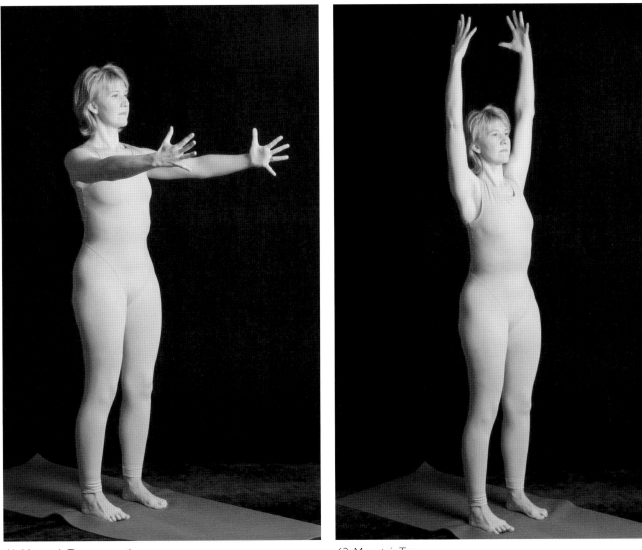

61 Mountain Top preparation

62 Mountain Top

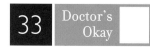

RIGHT ANGLE
Modified Adho Mukha Svanasana

Stretching out in Right Angle is a delicious way to release tension in your back, especially after you've been sitting or lying down for a long time.

benefits
Stretches hamstrings, calves, chest and back, tones abdomen

how to set up
Stand in Mountain about three feet away from a wall. Energize your feet and legs as in Mountain (p. 88).

Face the wall and take your hands to your hip creases. With your knees slightly bent, hinge forward over your hands, from where the tops of your thighs meet the front of your pelvis. Place your palms on the wall. Reach your hips back away from the wall so that your torso begins to come parallel to the ground. Walk your feet back so that they line up under your hips.

Draw the head of your arm bones deep into their shoulder joints. Now enliven your arms: reach out from the center of your chest and upper back as if you could press your palms straight through the wall (photo 63).

on your inhalations
With slightly bent knees, sweep your inner thighs back and wide as you did in Mountain. Slide your hips back, away from the wall, so that you feel less pressure on your wrist joints and instead shift more of your weight onto your legs. These actions will also lengthen your spine.

on your exhalations
Lightly draw your belly back toward your spine so that your abdomen feels strong and your lower back feels expansive and buoyant toward the sky, just as you did in Plank (p. 80). In this pose, if your spine is long (rather than hunched, rounded or swayed) and you can comfortably straighten your legs, then also dive your tailbone down, like an arrow shooting toward the earth. These actions will stabilize your lower body.

to intensify
Walk your hands down the wall, in line with your hips, so that your torso creates a right angle to your legs (photo 64).

Look at your hands: are your palms flat with fingers spread wide and middle fingers pointing directly up? Press more strongly into the wall with the thumb side of your hands. Spin your biceps up toward the sky and triceps down toward the earth. These actions will draw your arm bones even more deeply into your shoulder joints, create more space between your shoulders and ears, and strengthen your upper back.

to finish
Walk your feet in toward the wall and come back to standing in Mountain. Rest as needed, then continue on to Forward Fold.

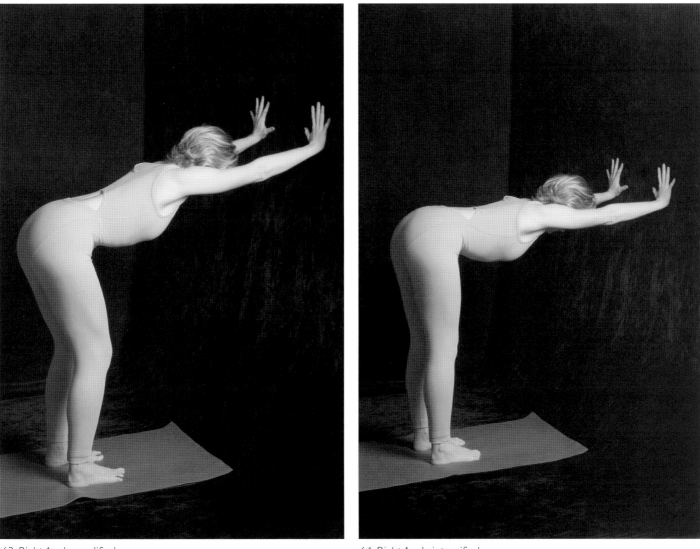

63 Right Angle modified

64 Right Angle intensified

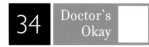
FORWARD FOLD
Modified Uttanasana

The strong foundation of powerful feet and legs in this pose feels, to me, like standing in my own truth and self-respect. The bow forward is with a regal, long spine and lifted heart, symbolically honoring myself and others.

benefits
Stretches hamstrings, calves, and back

how to set up
Stand with your back to a wall, your feet hips' width apart, and your feet twelve to eighteen inches away from the wall. Reach your hips back so that your buttocks press against the wall. As in Right Angle, take your hands to your hip creases and fold over your hands, right where the tops of your thighs meet the front of your pelvis. If your back rounds, bend your knees so that you can lengthen your spine. Keep your head in line with the rest of your spine (photo 65) rather than dropping your head down like a drooping flower.

on your inhalations
Notice that with full, rich inhalations, your torso floats up toward the sky half an inch or so.

on your exhalations
Bow with dignity. Keep your legs and torso long, as if they were blades of scissors drawing together. Keep your feet and toes energized and bright.

Notice if your shoulders are hunching. If so, lightly shrug your shoulders up in the direction of your ears, strongly roll the head of your arm bones back in the direction of the sky, and press your shoulder blades onto your back.

to intensify
Now extend your arms parallel to your legs, palms facing one another and fingers wide (photo 66).

to finish
Soften your knees and slowly roll up to standing in Mountain. Rest as needed, then continue on to Tree.

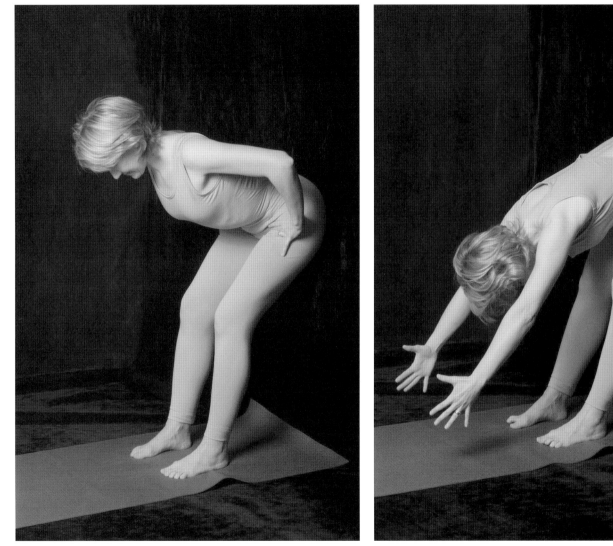

65 Forward Fold modified

66 Forward Fold intensified

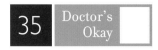
TREE

Vrksasana

Think of a magnificent tree during a wind and rain storm. Branches get whipped around and leaves torn off, but the tree's solid trunk and deep roots stay firmly grounded. In Tree, the steadfastness of your standing leg and core body support you as you expand upward and outward with your arms, like leafy branches reaching toward the light.

benefits

Strengthens legs and core body, opens hips and inner thighs, develops balance

how to set up

Stand in Mountain with the back of your body close to a wall. Take your hands to your hip creases. Shift your weight slightly onto your left leg and lengthen your spine upward. Turn your right knee out to the right. Place your right heel on your left ankle, with your right toes on the ground, so that you balance on your left foot (photo 67). If your balance feels unsteady today, lean back lightly against the wall.

on your inhalations

Breathe deeply into the circumference of your ribcage—to the front, the back, and the sides of your ribcage. Imagine inhaling the rich, damp air of a forest after a rainstorm. Draw this verdant energy into every cell of your body.

on your exhalations

Like a great tree sending down roots, extend down into the earth through your tailbone, left leg, and foot. This will create a rebounding action of your spine lengthening up toward the sky. Press your right thigh back in the direction of the wall behind you to find a gentle stretch in your right inner thigh.

to intensify

Sneak your right foot up to your left inner knee, or use your hands to bring your right foot up to your left inner thigh. Press your foot against your thigh, and press your thigh back against your foot. As in Mountain Top (p. 90), extend your arms overhead. Even as you reach toward the sky with your fingertips, remember to keep the head of your arm bones drawn deeply into their shoulder joints so that the top of your shoulders stay relaxed and down away from your ears (photo 68).

to finish

Slowly release your arms and right foot down. Rest in Mountain as needed, then try the pose on the second side. Continue on to Warrior I.

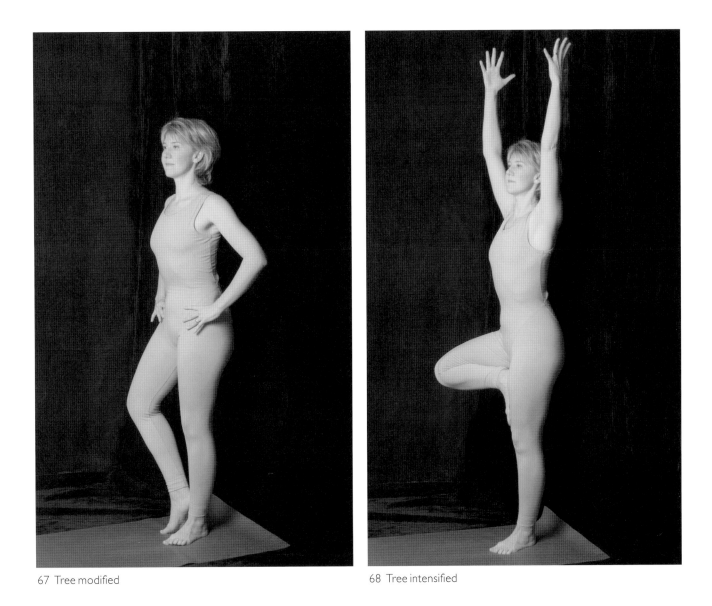

67 Tree modified

68 Tree intensified

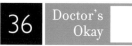

WARRIOR I
Modified Virabhadrasana I

To stay in this advanced version of Seated Warrior I (p. 34) for several breaths requires willpower. Every inhale, dig deep into your inner strength. Every exhale, commit to expressing yourself fully and radiantly.

benefits
Strengthens legs, chest and back, stretches hips and calves

how to set up
Stand in Mountain with your back at a wall. Step your right foot forward two to three feet, in line with your right hip. Bend your right knee so that your thigh begins to come parallel to the earth and your knee lines up over—not forward of—your right ankle. Press your left heel back against the wall. Take your hands on your hips and stand tall. Roll the head of your arm bones back and press your shoulder blades firmly onto your back (photo 69).

on your inhalations
Stabilize your pelvis: draw your right leg back and left leg forward to seat your thigh bones more deeply into their hip sockets.

on your exhalations
Keep that solidity, and now extend out fully: slide your right knee forward and press your left heel back.

to intensify
Boldly bend your right knee all the way into a right angle. Enthusiastically lift your left inner thigh up toward the sky.

Lightly shrug your shoulders up, strongly roll the head of your arm bones back, and press your shoulder blades onto your back. Extend your arms forward and overhead, and energize all the way out through your fingertips (photo 70). Stay steady in your *ujjayi* breath and grounded in your resolve.

to finish
Slowly release your arms down, straighten your front knee and step forward to stand in Mountain. Rest as needed, then try the pose on the second side. Continue on to Warrior II.

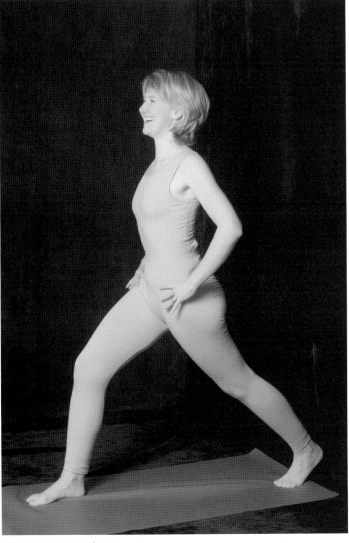

69 Warrior I modified

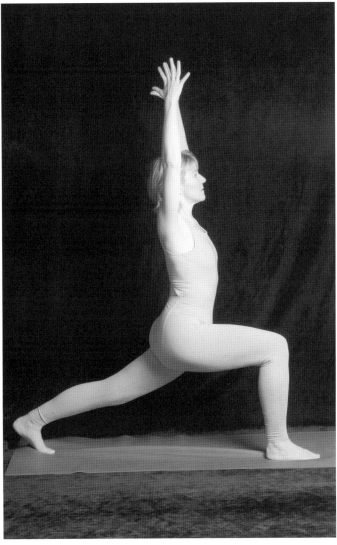

70 Warrior I intensified

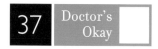

WARRIOR II
Virabhadrasana II

This is a pose with attitude! In Warrior II, you sink deeply into a lunge in your front leg, settling comfortably into your own power. You then turn a calm gaze ahead of you, over your front hand, ready to meet whatever comes your way.

benefits
Strengthens legs, back and abdomen, stretches inner thighs

how to set up
Facing away from the wall, stand close enough to the wall so that you can lean back against it if needed. Stand in Mountain. Step your feet wide, approximately the width of your outstretched arms. Turn your right foot parallel to the wall. Turn your left heel out, away from the midline of your body. Place your hands at your hip creases.

Bend your right knee so that your thigh begins to come parallel to the earth and your knee lines up over—not forward of—your right ankle. Keep your pelvis and torso facing the center of the room rather than facing toward your right leg. If your balance feels unsteady today, lean back lightly against the wall. Turn your head to look out over your right shoulder (photo 71).

As in Mountain (p. 88), sweep your inner thighs back and wide toward the wall behind you. Your buttocks may touch the wall. Then, even as you keep the back of your pelvis broad, anchor your tailbone toward the earth. These opposing actions bring your torso into the center of the power of the pose, enliven both legs, and lengthen your core body upward.

on your inhalations
Imagine filling every part of yourself with life energy, like a well filling up with sweet, clear water.

on your exhalations
Envision the well spilling over, an unending source of energy flowing through you and around you.

to intensify
Courageously sink the top of your right thigh down in line with your right knee. Resist your left inner thigh up toward the sky. Anchor down through the outside edge of your left foot.

From the center of your chest, powerfully extend your arms out, parallel to the ground. With soft eyes, gaze out beyond your right hand (photo 72).

to finish
Slowly release your arms, straighten your right knee, and step your feet together in Mountain. Rest as needed, then try the pose on the second side. Continue on to Triangle.

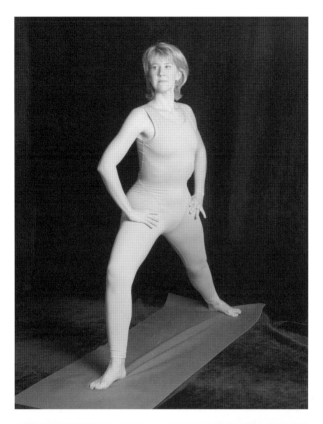

71 Warrior II modified

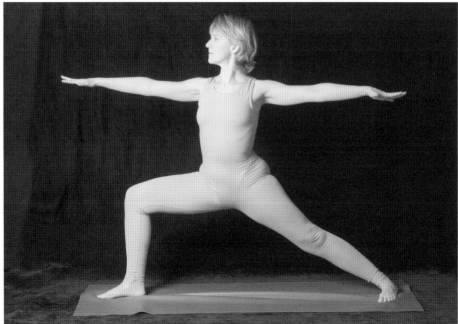

72 Warrior II intensified

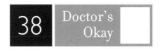
TRIANGLE
Utthita Trikonasana

To me, Triangle embodies courageously opening to life. Standing on the strong foundation of your legs, you lengthen your torso, open your arms wide, and reveal your shining heart.

I hope that you have experienced the receiving and giving of profound love at some time in your life. Even if your beloved is no longer here, the love you felt remains real. What if love were an essence you could draw into every cell of your body?

benefits
Strengthens legs, back, and abdomen, stretches sides of torso

how to set up
Facing away from the wall, stand close enough to the wall so that you can lean back against it if needed. Stand in Mountain. Step your feet wide, approximately the width of your outstretched arms. Turn your right foot parallel to the wall. Turn your left heel out, away from the midline of your body. Place your hands at your hip creases. Shift your hips to the left. As you do so, you will feel your right hip crease deepen underneath your right hand and your torso will come parallel to the ground. Rest your right hand onto your shin or a yoga block, and gaze down (photo 73). If your balance feels unsteady today, lean back lightly against the wall.

Just as in Warrior II (p. 100), sweep your inner thighs back and wide toward the wall behind you. Your buttocks may touch the wall. Then, even as you keep the back of your pelvis broad, powerfully anchor your tailbone toward the earth. These opposing actions will bring your torso into alignment over your front leg, enliven both legs, and lengthen your core body.

on your inhalations
Imagine saturating yourself with love.

on your exhalations
Now imagine emanating love all around you, like heat rising off your skin.

to intensify
When your core body feels long and strong, on your exhales turn your belly and heart upward. From the center of your chest and back, extend your left arm up toward the sky and extend energy down through your right arm toward the earth (photo 74). Glance down—has your torso curled forward of your front leg? If so, take your bottom hand high enough on a yoga block or your front leg so that you can elongate your spine and bring your torso and head in line with your front leg.

to finish
Slowly float your torso back upright, release your arms, and step your feet together in Mountain. Rest as needed, then try the pose on the second side. Continue on to Half Moon.

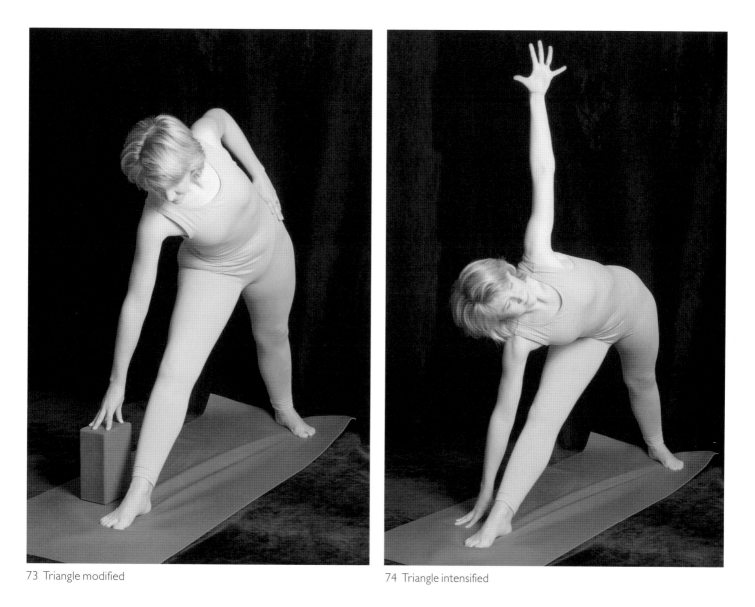

73 Triangle modified

74 Triangle intensified

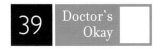
HALF MOON
Ardha Chandrasana

Our last strength and stamina-building pose is an advanced version of Seated Half Moon (p. 30). This pose embodies the rootedness of Tree, the expansiveness of Triangle, and the courageousness of balancing. When it all comes together, Half Moon feels like flying!

benefits
Strengthens legs, back and abdomen, stretches hamstrings and calves

how to set up
In this version of Half Moon, you will come into Triangle to the right (p. 102), lean back lightly on the wall behind you if needed, and then shift forward to stand on your right foot. Before you come into the pose, you may wish to set up a yoga block about twelve inches in front of your right foot.

From Triangle, rest your left hand onto your hip and look down at your right foot. Bend your right knee and begin to shift forward to stand on your right leg (photo 75). Press your right fingertips onto the block or the ground. Take a small step forward with your left foot, then, lead from the power of your core body to float your left leg up toward the sky. You may wish to rest the back of your head and your left heel on the wall behind you. Stack your left hip directly over your right hip. One or both buttocks may rest on the wall. Spin your belly and chest upward as you gaze down.

on your inhalations
Imagine inhaling bright energy.

on your exhalations
Shine out like a bright moon floating in the night sky. Invite your body to become more alive and expansive in all directions.

to intensify
Glance down at your right leg and make sure your knee lines up directly over your foot. Energize both legs. Strongly flex your left foot. Revolve your torso upward. If your left shoulder lines up over your right shoulder, it will be comfortable to extend your left arm toward the sky. If not, keep your left hand on your left waist. Float your left leg higher, in line with your left hip. Gaze down or forward (photo 76).

to finish
Slowly step your left foot down, float your torso back upright, release your arms, and step your feet together in Mountain. Rest as needed, then try the pose on the second side. Continue on to Rag Doll.

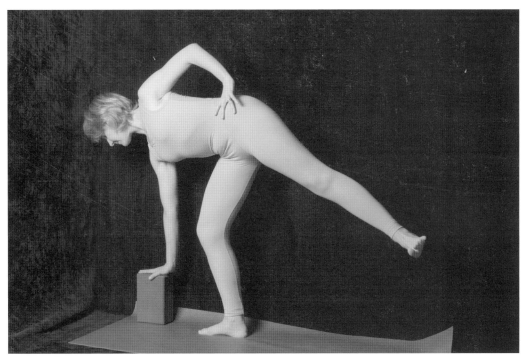

75 Half Moon modified

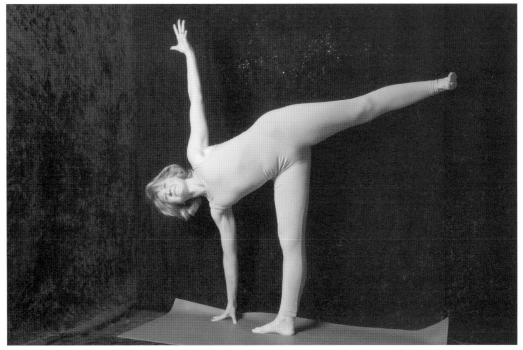

76 Half Moon intensified

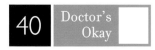
RAG DOLL
Modified Uttanasana

After practicing the robust standing poses, your body will be ready to receive the gift of rest. Rag Doll is a wonderful passive stretch for your back that will ease you into Resting Pose.

benefits
Releases tension in shoulders and back

how to set up
From Mountain, soften your knees and roll down through your spine. Hold your opposite elbows with your hands. Let your head and arms hang down (photo 77). Imagine your body as heavy and soft as a wet rag doll hung out to dry over a clothesline. If your balance feels unsteady today, rest your buttocks against the wall behind you.

on your inhalations
You may notice a subtle expansion and lift of your back body on your inhalations. Let your face relax totally.

on your exhalations
Allow your body to have weight and softness.

to finish
Release your arms and creep down slowly onto all fours, then into Resting Child (p. 44) for a few breaths. Finally, roll onto your back and stretch out in Resting Pose (p. 19). Please make yourself comfortable and savor this deep relaxation for five to ten minutes.

* * *

As your stamina increases, you might enjoy linking the poses together into a smooth flow. Like a butterfly easily floating from blossom to blossom, please luxuriate in each pose for a few long breaths, then transition to the next pose in slow motion. Here is a sample sequence to play with:

MOUNTAIN: Stand in Mountain

TREE: Shift onto your right foot and come into Tree, left foot up

WARRIOR I: In slow motion, bend your right knee into a right angle as you step your left foot way back into Warrior I

WARRIOR II: Keep your right knee bent, open your arms wide, and turn your pelvis and torso open into Warrior II

TRIANGLE: Straighten your right knee and shift your hips to the left to come into Triangle to the right

HALF MOON: Take a small step forward with your left foot, then blossom into Half Moon standing on your right foot

TRIANGLE: In slow motion, bend your right knee and touch your left foot back down again into Triangle

MOUNTAIN: Float your torso upright again and step into Mountain

Rest as needed, then try the sequence on the second side.

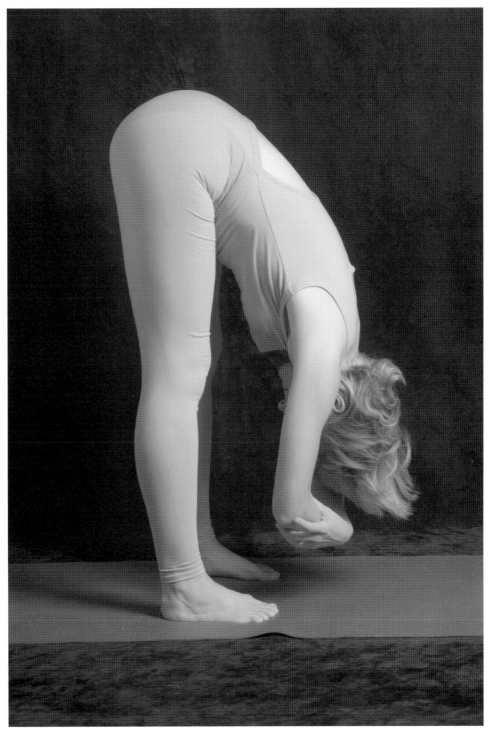

77 Rag Doll

Following are descriptions and pictures of the anatomical landmarks referred to in this book.

Your **pelvis** is the bowl-shaped bony structure of your hips. Your two hips are comprised of ilium, ischium, and pubic bones. Like two halves of a bowl, these bones mirror one another on the left and right sides of your body (photos 78 and 79).

Your left and right hip bones connect at the front of your body at your **pubic bones** located just above your genitals (photos 78 and 79).

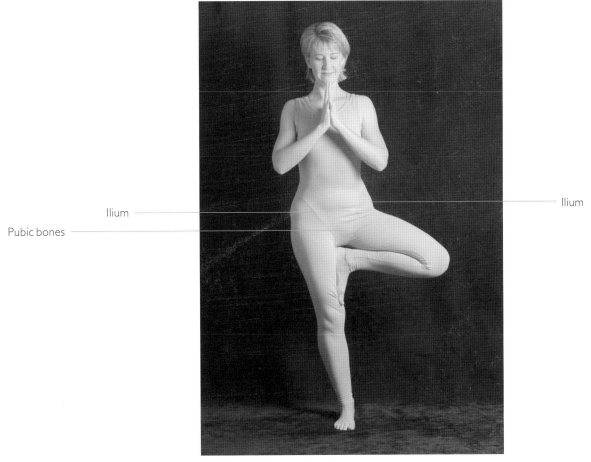

Ilium

Pubic bones

Ilium

78 Tree

To find your **sit bones**, sit on an unpadded chair or uncarpeted floor and tilt the front of your pelvis forward as in Seated Mountain preparation. You will feel the pressure of two bony bumps (the ischial tuberosities that are at the base of your left and right ischium) into the chair or ground (photos 79 and 80).

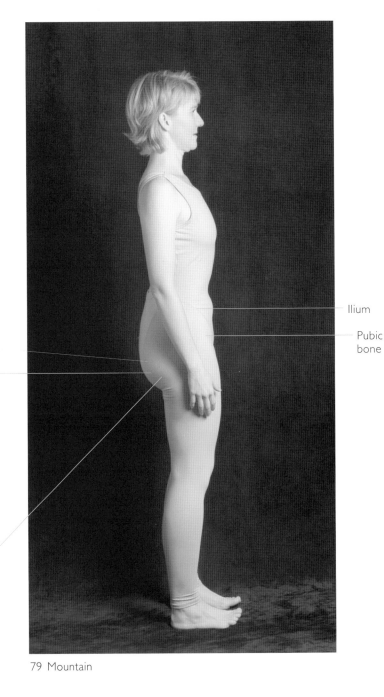

Ilium

Pubic bone

Ischium

Sit bones

Tailbone

79 Mountain

Here, you can also feel your **hip creases**. Press your hands into the creases between where the tops of your thighs meet the front of your hips. In most yoga poses, you will hinge forward at your hip creases (photo 80).

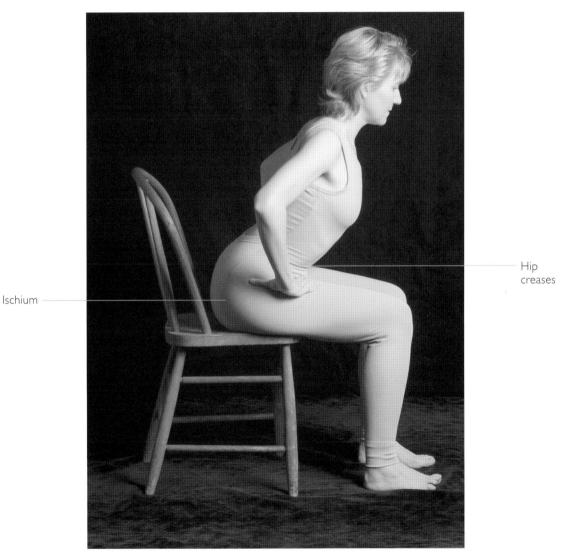

Ischium

Hip creases

80 Seated Mountain preparation

To find your **tailbone**, now round through your spine as in Seated Cat. The pressure on your sit bones goes away as you roll off your sit bones and onto your last vertebrae. (Your vertebrae are the column of bones that make up your spine.) The last of the four main sections of vertebrae of your spine also comprise your sacrum, which connects to the left and right back sides of your hip bones via sacroiliac joints. Your tailbone is made up of the very last vertebrae that curve in slightly toward the front of your body like a crooked finger (photos 79 and 81).

To find the **head of your arm bone**, place one

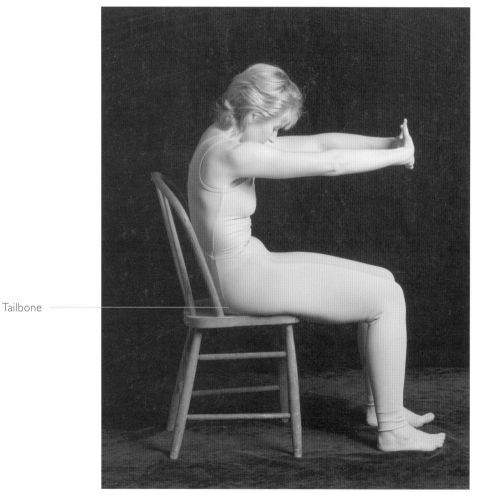

Tailbone

81 Seated Cat

hand on your opposite outer shoulder. This is where the articular head of the humerus bone fits into the glenoid cavity within the scapula. In plain language, you are touching the top of your upper arm bone, close to the knobby top of the bone that fits into a shallow bowl-shaped indentation within your shoulder blade. Several muscles create stability and movement of the head of your arm bone in its shoulder joint (photo 82).

The instruction to "lightly shrug the head of

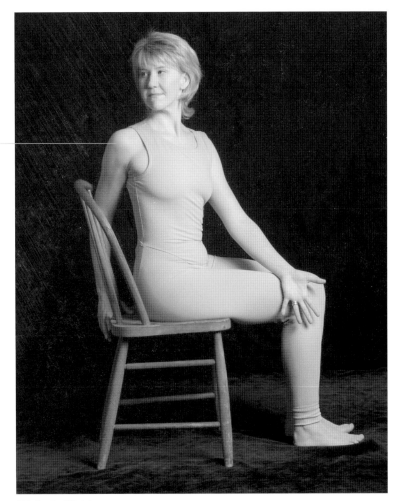

Head of the arm bone

82 Seated Twist

your arm bones up and back" is to help you find movement in the bony structure of your shoulder girdle (shoulder blades, collarbones, breastbone, head of your arm bones) and their supporting muscles—all without clenching the tops of your shoulders up toward your ears.

To find the **four corners of your feet**, sit comfortably in a chair. Cross your right ankle above your right knee, as in Seated Half Lotus Preparation.

Use your hands to massage the sole of your right foot and to find the mound of your big toe, mound of your little toe, inner heel, and outer heel (photo 83).

Do the same massage for your left foot. Now stand barefoot on an uncarpeted floor to sense the same four corners of your feet that you were just massaging in contact with the ground.

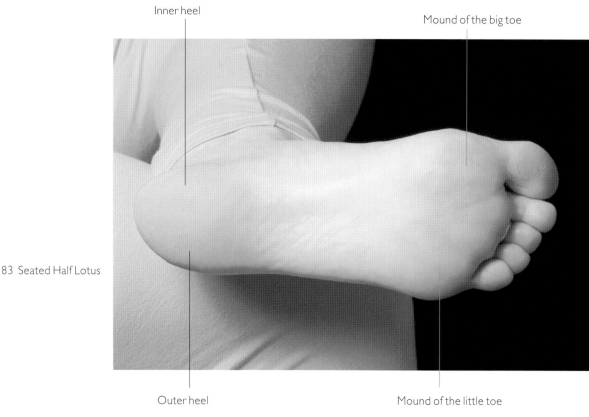

Inner heel

Mound of the big toe

83 Seated Half Lotus

Outer heel

Mound of the little toe

RESOURCES

yoga equipment

Hugger-Mugger Yoga Products
800-473-4888
www.huggermugger.com

Living Arts
800-2-LIVING
www.livingarts.com

where to find a yoga teacher

Anusara Yoga
Teacher Directory
www.anusarayoga.com

Yoga Journal Magazine
Teacher Directory
www.yogajournal.com

books on yoga

Back Care Basics
Mary Pullig Schatz, M.D.
Berkeley, CA: Rodmell Press, 1992

The Breathing Book: Good Health and Vitality through Essential Breath Work
Donna Farhi
New York, NY: Owl Books, 1996

Relax and Renew: Restful Yoga for Stressful Times
Judith Lasater, Ph.D., P.T.
Berkeley, CA: Rodmell Press, 1995

Yoga: The Spirit and Practice of Moving into Stillness
Erich Schiffmann
New York, NY: Pocket Books, 1996

yoga videos / cds

Anusara Yoga 101

John Friend, double-cd set

888-398-9642

www.anusara.com

River of Devotion: Anusara Yoga with Sarahjoy Marsh

Double-cd set

(503) 552-YOGA

www.yogajoy.net

Yoga Alignment and Form

John Friend, video

www.anusara.com

***Yoga Journal*'s Yoga Practice Series**

Videos

www.yogajournal.com

living with cancer

American Cancer Society

1-800-227-2345 (GA)

www.cancer.org

Includes *Reach for Recovery*, the ACS rehabilitation program for women and men with breast cancer to help with physical, emotional, and cosmetic needs related to the cancer and treatment side effects.

CancerCare, Inc.

1-800-813-4673 (NY)

www.cancercare.org

Free professional emotional support, information, financial assistance, and practical help by oncology social workers.

Cancer Hope Network

1-877-467-3638 (NJ)

www.cancerhopenetwork.org

One-to-one support from survivors.

Cancer Information and Counseling Line

1-800-525-3777 (CO)

www.amc.org

Service for cancer survivors, family members, and friends, the general public of medical information and emotional support through short-term counseling, and resource referrals.

Cancer Information Service

1-800-4-CANCER (9 AM–4:30 PM, local time)

www.cancer.gov (LiveHelp, 9 AM–10 PM Eastern Time)

The program of the National Cancer Institute to communicate the latest research-based information in understandable language to patients, families, medical professionals, and the general public.

Cancer Lifeline

1-800-255-5505 24-Hour Lifeline (WA)

www.cancerlifeline.org

Provides emotional support about cancer-related issues via 24-Hour Lifeline. Offers a wide range of programs, support groups, classes, and presentations aimed at optimizing the quality of life for cancer patients, cancer survivors and their families, friends, co-workers, and caregivers.

Encore Plus

1-800-953-7587 (NY)

or local YWCA www.ywca.org

YWCA discussion and exercise program for breast cancer surgical patients.

Gilda's Club

1-888-445-3248 (NY)

www.gildasclub.org

Social and emotional support to cancer patients, their families, and friends through lectures, workshops, classes, and other events.

Living Beyond Breast Cancer

1-888-753-5222 (PA)

www.lbbc.org

Helpline and programs with support for quality of life for breast cancer patients and survivors.

National Lymphedema Network

1-800-541-3259 (CA)

www.lymphnet.org

Information on prevention and treatment of lymphedema.

Y-ME (Breast Cancer Support Groups)

1-800-221-2141 (IL)

www.y-me.org

Pre-surgery counseling, treatment information, peer support for breast cancer patients.

INDEX OF POSES